Nina Musurlieva

Chronic periodontitis. Risk factors, quality of life

Nina Musurlieva

Chronic periodontitis. Risk factors, quality of life

LAP LAMBERT Academic Publishing

Impressum / Imprint

Bibliografische Information der Deutschen Nationalbibliothek: Die Deutsche Nationalbibliothek verzeichnet diese Publikation in der Deutschen Nationalbibliografie; detaillierte bibliografische Daten sind im Internet über http://dnb.d-nb.de abrufbar.

Alle in diesem Buch genannten Marken und Produktnamen unterliegen warenzeichen-, marken- oder patentrechtlichem Schutz bzw. sind Warenzeichen oder eingetragene Warenzeichen der jeweiligen Inhaber. Die Wiedergabe von Marken, Produktnamen, Gebrauchsnamen, Handelsnamen, Warenbezeichnungen u.s.w. in diesem Werk berechtigt auch ohne besondere Kennzeichnung nicht zu der Annahme, dass solche Namen im Sinne der Warenzeichen- und Markenschutzgesetzgebung als frei zu betrachten wären und daher von jedermann benutzt werden dürften.

Bibliographic information published by the Deutsche Nationalbibliothek: The Deutsche Nationalbibliothek lists this publication in the Deutsche Nationalbibliografie; detailed bibliographic data are available in the Internet at http://dnb.d-nb.de.

Any brand names and product names mentioned in this book are subject to trademark, brand or patent protection and are trademarks or registered trademarks of their respective holders. The use of brand names, product names, common names, trade names, product descriptions etc. even without a particular marking in this work is in no way to be construed to mean that such names may be regarded as unrestricted in respect of trademark and brand protection legislation and could thus be used by anyone.

Coverbild / Cover image: www.ingimage.com

Verlag / Publisher:
LAP LAMBERT Academic Publishing
ist ein Imprint der / is a trademark of
OmniScriptum GmbH & Co. KG
Heinrich-Böcking-Str. 6-8, 66121 Saarbrücken, Deutschland / Germany
Email: info@lap-publishing.com

Herstellung: siehe letzte Seite /
Printed at: see last page
ISBN: 978-3-659-39763-9

Zugl. / Approved by: Plovdiv, Medical University Plovdiv, 2013

Copyright © 2015 OmniScriptum GmbH & Co. KG
Alle Rechte vorbehalten. / All rights reserved. Saarbrücken 2015

Chronic periodontitis.

Risk factors, quality of life

Nina M. Musurlieva DDS, PhD

Department of Social Medicine and Public Health, Faculty of Public Health,

Medical University of Plovdiv, Bulgaria

Content

Introduction	3
1. Risk factors for development of chronic periodontitis	4
1.1. Etiologic factors	5
1.2. Determinants of risk	6
1.3. Systematic risk factors	8
1.4. Systemic risk indicators	13
1.5. Own study	15
2. Quality of life	23
2.1. Aspects of the impact of periodontitis on the quality of life	25
2.2. Tools for assessment of the impact of oral health on quality of life	27
2.3. Assessment of the impact of periodontitis on the quality of life in the own research	33
Conclusion	42
References	44

Introduction

Periodontal diseases have been known since ancient times. Paleostomatology is the science that studies the dental organs and tissues of prehistoric people. It indicates the presence of chronic periodontal changes even in remnants of pre-Neanderthal mandibles. The library of the king of Assyria, Ashurbanipal, is full of recipes for treatment of periodontal diseases. Such were found in ancient Iberian papyri, and their symptoms were even described in detail in writings of physicians from the time of the Chou dynasty. As ancient the periodontal diseases are, as old is the ambition of people to restore their lost teeth due to them. In Honduras a skull of the pre-Colombian era was discovered, in which a cutter was found carved from stone and attached to the bone. Thousands of years ago in Egypt intraosseous implantation of teeth from ivory was made in the jaws of courtly ladies, menaced with the absence of front teeth.

Periodontitis affects the tissues surrounding and supporting the teeth in their alveoli leading to inflammation and recession of the gum, a formation of periodontal pockets, resorption of alveolar bone. The last two symptoms lead to increased mobility of teeth, baring and migration, periodontal abscesses and tooth loss. In patients with Periodontitis a change has been seen in the functions - speech and chewing, which creates health problems from the eating difficulty and the emergence of a number of common diseases.

Numerous studies prove that Periodontitis has a negative impact on the quality of life, affecting its main aspects - physical, social, psychological well-being and social activity of the individual. Parodontitis is the main reason for edentulism of the population globally - a problem with high social value.

The loss of teeth leads to psychological trauma in the patient, equivalent to the loss of any other organ. The lack of teeth affects the emotional state by inducing shame in the individual and attempt to conceal the state as a result of the impaired aesthetics. Limited social activity has been observed. All these facts point to a direct link between periodontitis and the quality of life of the patient.

The monograph discusses the problems of patients with chronic periodontitis, their quality of life, the risk factors for developing the disease have been revealed.

Today Periodontitis is one the most common oral diseases. The worldwide prevalence of periodontal diseases is 5-20% in the adult population. Periodontitis is the second largest oral health problem, affecting 10-15% of the world's population [1]. The most severe forms of periodontal disease significantly affect adults 35-44 years old with a prevalence of 19%. Europeans aged 35-44 are with 13-54% small differences for Eastern Europe (45%) and Western (36%). In a US study of 2002 Brown et al. reported that 33% of the cases ended up with loss of lever of 5 mm, and 8% were with severe periodontitis [2].

According to American Academia of Periodontology, chronic periodontitis is more prevalent in adults; the amount of bone loss is compatible with local characteristics; subgingival calculus is a common finding; and the disease usually has slow to moderate progression [3]. Based on the continuously changing concepts about periodontal diseases in recent years, American Academia of Periodontology has proposed different classifications. In 1985, Page and Schroeder described in their work "about periodontitis in humans and other animals" the different types of periodontitis. Based on their studies, in 1989 at Word Workshop it was assumed that periodontitis of adults is typical for patients over 35 with slow flowing horizontal bone resorption. In 1999 Word Workshop the name periodontitis of adults was changed to periodontitis chronica [2].

Chronic periodontitis has been further classified as localized or generalized depending on whether <30% or >30% of sites are involved. Severity is based on the amount of clinical attachment (CAL) loss and is designated as slight (1-2 mm CAL), moderate (3-4 mm CAL) or severe (>5mm CAL).

Risk factors for development of periodontitis

The detection of risk factors for the occurrence of periodontitis is complicated. In most cases it is necessary to have more of them, in order to distort the immune responses of the organism. Often different ways of combining between several risk factors have been observed, ranging during the different stages of the life of the organism [4].

Periodontitis is a disease with multifactorial etiology. Main etiological factor for its development is the bacterial plaque. Not all plaque deposits lead to the development of periodontal disease, not every untreated gingivitis causes periodontal destruction [5].

These facts impose the notion of the existence of factors different from the plaque, changing the protective response of the organism to the periodontal infection and determining its susceptibility to it. Robert Genco and Valerie Clerehugh distinguish two large groups of RF for periodontitis:

1. Local - wrongly made restorations, thickening of the teeth, breathing through the mouth, muscle parafunctions, quantity and composition of the saliva, mechanical,

thermal, chemical and radiation disabilities, etc. [6] 2. Systemic factors - smoking, diabetes, genetic abnormalities, stress, systemic diseases, AIDS, intake of medications, poor diet, age, sex, education, socioeconomic status, etc. [6]. In the combination of external factors such as smoking, medications, stress, malnutrition the systemic neuroendocrine-immunological mechanisms, building the protection of the microorganism, can be modified [7]. Other systemic factors such as sex, age, race, affect the progression of the periodontal disease in the individual or in specific groups. [8] According to these authors, there are the so called risk indicators (potential risk factors) for the development of periodontal diseases such as obesity, osteoporosis, low calcium levels, osteopenia, which presence is associated with an increased chance of developing a disease [6]. In the opinion of a group of Spanish scientists [9] to the following groups a third one is added - determinants of risk. In it they separate age, sex, socio-economic status.

1.1. Etiologic factors for development of periodontitis
Impact of dental plaque in the etiology of periodontitis

Periodontal diseases have infectious nature [10,11]. Dental plaque microorganisms [6,10-13] are accepted as a major etiologic factor triggering pathological processes in periodontitis. The idea of the infectious beginning has evolved over the years. For 60 years the authors have accepted it as the only sufficient for the development of the disease, but later, their concept has been replaced by a more balanced bacterial-immunological theory of the etiology of inflammatory periodontal diseases. According to it, the plaque is required for the development of periodontitis, but is not sufficient for the occurrence of the disease [6]. The disease incidence is largely dependent on the protective factors of macroorganisms [11,14]. The quantity of plaque is determined by the level of oral care of the individual.

Many epidemiological studies showed a causal relationship between the severity of periodontal disease and the two mentioned factors [10,11].

In 1959 Schei et al. tracked in 737 people the level of oral hygiene and the degree of periodontal damage. They found statistically reliable positive correlation: the more poor oral hygiene, the more severe are the periodontal impairments [15]. Other scientists have pointed out that the correlation between poor oral hygiene and periodontal condition is so close to the linear, that it can only be compared with the correlation periodontal disease - age [16,17].

Role of subgingival calculus in the etiology of periodontal diseases

For five millennia calculus has been considered as the main etiological factor for periodontal diseases [18]. This view was changed during the 60s of this century as a result of numerous experimental studies and detection of the infectious onset of periodontitis.

Epidemiological studies have shown a close relationship between calculus and periodontal pathogens [18,19]. There is no evidence for its role as the primary cause of their development. Tartar affects the development of dental plaque - on it food and toxins are deposited that alter the bacterial ecosystem and its growth maintain the plaque near the tissues [19]. In this aspect it contributes to the chronic inflammation and progression of the disease [6]. There are no studies evaluating the effect of treatment of periodontal pathogens without removing the tartar [19].

1.2. Determinants of risk for periodontitis
Impact of age factor on the incidence of periodontitis

Opinions whether with aging the risk of developing periodontal diseases increases, are contradictory. According to some authors persons who reached old age are "resilient" and less prone to periodontitis [20]. The likelihood of developing periodontitis is small, as these persons have already been exposed to the risk of the disease at a younger age [21].

There is no clear justification whether aging of the individual is associated with a higher periodontal incidence. There is no direct correlation between the two processes, if the oral hygiene of the people surveyed is good throughout their life [18,22]. Such evidence was presented by Burt and Abdellatif. In their longitudinal study they reached the conclusion that age does not play a role as a risk factor for the appearance of periodontitis, if during all his/her life the individual has maintained good oral hygiene [23].

The magnitude of the risk of disease is determined by calculating the relative risk (odds ratio). In one case, for exposure the poor oral hygiene is used, and in the second - age. The risk of periodontitis in people with poor oral hygiene is 20.52, while in people who have passed adulthood is only 1.24.

Proof of the causal connection based on evidence on the impact of age on the development of periodontitis, is associated with many problems. One of them is that with aging the systemic illness in the individual increase too, and they in their turn are also a risk factor for periodontitis. Their accumulation, rather than the susceptibility of the individual, is the reason for prevalence of periodontitis in this age group [24]. For the conduction of epidemiological studies it is not possible to isolate a real old group of individuals. First, because of gaps in the definition of the concept itself, and second, the lack of a single opinion of the authors, over how many years individuals are actually adults [25]. For these reasons, most authors associate aging with biological and microbiological changes occurring in periodontium [18,26]. Some authors define it as an associated factor for periodontitis [27]. In the literature prevailing is the view that older people (who have passed adulthood) suffer more often and more severe forms of periodontitis. Chronic periodontitis is associated with adult patients (in earlier classifications it is called periodontitis of adulthood) [6,18,22]. A study conducted by George Taylor in the USA a correlation is made between age and severity of periodontitis. It was found that in the age group 55-64 predominate are the moderate and severe forms of periodontitis - 71.79%, as opposed to the group of 18-29 year olds. They are 21.60% and there dominant are the mild forms of periodontitis - 89.22% [28]. Severe periodontitis with heavy loss of attachment over 7 mm is the most common cause of tooth loss [18,29]. Given the trend of aging of the population worldwide [1.31] determined can be the social significance of these diseases and the special care required by people who have passed adulthood, for improvement of their quality of life [14,18,30,31].

Impact of sex, race, education, socio-economic status of the individual on the prevalence of periodontitis
Sex:

Studies of a number of authors - Sheiham, Russell, Waerhaug, Yaneva, Andreeva prove that periodontal damage affect more often men than women. In men a higher incidence of periodontal disease with the formation of pockets is observed [4]. The male sex is defined as a systematic risk factor for the appearance of periodontitis, which according to some authors is associated with the poor oral hygiene [6,18]. When comparing men and women of the same age group, with equal oral hygiene, no the difference in the incidence of Periodontitis is proved [18].

Race:

The studies NHANES 1999-2000, NHANES 2001-2002, NHANES 2003-2004, conducted in the USA, show that the development of periodontal diseases affect the race, the type of education and socio-economic status of the individuals studied [32]. Their data suggest that the relative risk of developing periodontitis is much higher in black people, in people with low economic income and without higher education, compared to white people, with high annual income and good education. Black people are 2.66 times more prone to develop periodontal disease than white people. If the race factor is associated with the factors education and socio-economic status, black people show 1.94 (95% guaranteed probability) times higher risk for the occurrence of periodontal disease [32]. Such are the results from the epidemiological study of the University of Michigan for social studies. People who are not Caucasians suffer from more severe forms of periodontitis. Persons with higher education and income show a lower incidence of the disease [28]. In the study at the University of Adelaide the highest annual income of the people studied is considered as a stimulating factor for good oral health [33]. The influence of these socio-economic indicators can not be considered in isolation. They are usually associated with demographic factors - sex, age, marital status, number of visits to the dentist, as well as the systemic risk factors - diabetes, smoking.

1.3. Systemic risk factors for the development of periodontitis
Effect of smoking on the frequency and severity of periodontal diseases

In literature available are multiple data on the importance of the use of tobacco on the development, frequency, severity of the periodontal disease and the loss of teeth [34-41]. Smoking is one of the most important factors for the development of periodontitis [6,22,42,43]. The evidence for its role as a prevalent risk factor is follows: 1. A higher frequency of the disease among smokers than non-smokers in sectional studies. 2. A higher risk of occurrence of periodontal disease among smokers in conducting longitudinal studies 3. Statistically established significant association when compared with other risk factors [22]. Numerous studies prove that among smokers there are more severe forms of periodontitis with deep pockets, significant loss of attachment and alveolar bone [44-46].

The mechanisms of the effects of smoking have been studied in detail. Some authors consider that smokers have a reduced oral hygiene, higher accumulation of plaque and tartar, which leads to difference in the microbial flora in comparison to non-smokers. There the periodontal pockets are with anaerobic environment that supports the growth of anaerobic gram-negative periodontal pathogens [47,48]. Most studies show the opposite, that there is an insignificant difference in the level of plaque accumulation between the two groups [47]. There is no detectable difference in the levels of specific bacteria Porphyromonas gingivalis, Tannerella forsythia, Aggregatibacter actinomycetemcomitans in smokers and non-smokers [49].

In another study involving 798 people, it was reported that smokers have a significantly higher amount of Tannerella forsythia [50]. Since smoking has no significant effect on the bacterial flora, the scientists focused their attention on the mechanisms by which it affects the organism's immune response. On the one hand, tobacco products violate the normal ability to neutralize infections, on the other hand, they overstimulate the organism to degrades healthy tissue [47]. Smokers have reduced levels of antibodies in saliva Ig A and reduced serum Ig G antibody response to Prevotela intermedia Fusobacterium nukleatum [51]. Nicotine and its breakdown product cotinine are accumulated in crevicular fluid and saliva of smokers. Nicotine in high concentrations inhibits phagocytosis and leads to changes in the types of enzymes released by neutrophils [47]. This leads to distortion of the control of periodontal infections and damage of periodontal tissues. It has been established that nicotine can directly damage the cells of the periodontium - it is retained in fibroblasts by changing their morphology and prevents them from synthesizing collagen. Nicotine deposits on the root surface and impregnates it, which leads to impaired healing and tissue regeneration and compromise conventional periodontal treatment in smokers [6,47].

The relation periodontitis - smoking is very well demonstrated in NHANES 3 - Third National Health and Nutrition Servey, a study of 12,000 people over 18 years in the USA [49]. It was observed that in smokers periodontitis occurs four times more frequently than in non-smokers. This study demonstrates the relation dose - response between cigarettes smoked per day and the relative risk to develop a disease. Individuals smoking more than 31 cigarettes per day are six times more disposed to develop periodontitis. These data coincide with those obtained in other sectional studies in Europe and the USA - the relative risk in smokers to develop periodontitis varies from 1.5 to 7.3 depending on the severity of the disease [45]. The conclusion to be made is that smoking is a risk factor for the appearance of periodontitis. The influence of the long period of smoking and the amount of cigarettes smoked has been proved in adult patients. In younger patients (19 to 30) tobacco smoking is associated with increases of the severity of the generalized aggressive periodontitis [52]. Longitudinal studies have shown that in young smokers, consuming more than 15 cigarettes per day, the risk of teeth loss is greater [53]. The use of pipe has a similar effect of influence on periodontium with that of cigarettes [54].

Diabetes mellitus

Diabetes mellitus is an important system factor for the development of periodontitis. In people with diabetes the periodontal disease has a much higher prevalence and severity [6,22,55-57]. Periodontitis is considered the sixth complication of diabetes [63]. Study of Indians in the state of Arizona provides an extensive information on the correlation diabetes-periodontal disease [6]. Their community is characterized by a high frequency of non-insulin dependent type of diabetes. In all age groups diabetic patients have a higher frequency and severity of periodontal destruction [14]. In earlier studies, before 1980, the type of diabetes was not define in the study group of patients. Modern studies are based on the separation of the two types of diabetes, and the degree of metabolic control [52]. There are some data indicating that the severity of periodontal destruction may be related to the type of diabetes, the duration of disease, the level of metabolic control [59-61]. Patients with insulin-dependent diabetes (it occurs in young individuals) suffer longer and their risk for developing periodontitis is higher [10]. Cases with well-controlled diabetes are characterized by similar levels of periodontal destruction in comparison with those without diabetes [60-63]. In search of correlation between diabetes and periodontitis the following factors should be taken into account - sex, age, plaque and tartar, which can play the role of confounding factors. Only diabetic status, age and subgingival tartar are in significant correlation with the higher frequency and severity of periodontal diseases [18]. Between diabetes and periodontitis, there is two-way relation. Not only the diabetes is a risk factor for the occurrence of periodontal disease, but the infection of periodontal tissues itself can induce resistance of the tissues to insulin and lead to the onset of diabetes [60-68]. At the World Workshop in 1996 Offenbacher proposes to introduce a new concept – "periodontitis medicine" which reflects exactly this relation and emphasizes the collaboration between doctors and dentists [60]. Many epidemiological studies prove the bidirectional relation as its association can be demonstrated with the criteria of Bradford-Hill. Interesting is the study of Sanz Sanches and Bascones Martinez, making meta-analysis and systematic information according to each of the eleven criteria [65].

Genetic aspects of periodontal diseases

The role of heredity in the occurrence and development of periodontal disease is the most studied in recent years [6,69,70]. More than 100 syndromes aggravate periodontal diseases. Among them important are the genetically determined syndromes - Down syndrome, Papillon-Lefevre syndrome, Chediak-Higashi syndrome, lazy leucocyte syndrome [18]. The influence of genetic factors is different on different types of periodontitis and has been studied in each one of them [71]. There is sufficient scientific evidence on the role that genetic factors play in the development of aggressive periodontitis. Studies on twins have shown that in chronic periodontitis the role of heredity is variable and uncertain [72]. Genetic factors can have an influence during early onset of this form of periodontitis (in younger patients) [72]. There is an association between periodontitis and variation of certain genes (polymorphism) encoding various cytokines and inflammatory mediators involved in the pathogenesis of the disease [73]. It is believed that the polymorphism of the vitamin D receptor has been associated with the loss of alveolar bone. Beyond doubt was proven the familial tendency for a higher incidence of juvenile periodontitis [71]. On this basis, different genetic tests have been developed for risk assessment for the appearance of periodontitis.

Effects of other systemic diseases on periodontal diseases

The presence of systemic disease is associated with increased frequency and severity of periodontal diseases. Some authors examine the epidemiology of these diseases in correlation with gastro-intestinal, hepatic, neural, blood, blood-vessel diseases, collagen, etc. [18,74]. The relation systemic disease - periodontitis has not yet been objectively proven and refined [18]. Undoubtful is the fact that the violations in neutrophil function (in cyclic neutropenia, chronic neutropenia, etc.) lead to increased susceptibility of tissues to infection and periodontal destruction [75]. This factor plays a leading role in the pathogenesis of aggressive periodontitis. Studies have shown that 70-78% of patients with this diagnosis have impaired chemotaxis [76].

Impact of the acquired immune deficiency syndrome (AIDS) and HIV infection on periodontal diseases

Among the symptoms of HIV infected patients often it has been reported of oral manifestations. They are not caused by HIV per se, but appear secondary as a result of immunodepression [18]. HIV-infection and AIDS increase the risk of development of periodontitis and loss of atachment [77-79] Scientists have not yet reached a consensus on the classification and diagnosis of periodontal manifestations associated with HIV-infection [68]. In 1999, at Workshop International, it was assumed that HIV-infected patients may develop necrosis-ulcerative periodontitis and chronic periodontitis ongoing with rapid attachment degradation [68]. Patients with severe immunodeficiency not always develop severe periodontitis. This is explained by the frequent consumption of antibiotics [18]. It is difficult to establish the frequency of necrotic ulcerative periodontitis, due to the lack of consensus between the authors and the fact that it does not take into account the different medications taken by patients. One of the largest studies on this form of periodontitis involving 700 HIV infected patients reported a frequency of 6.3%. The same study showed a higher frequency of the disease among gay /bisexual men/ than in the other HIV-infected [81]. The impaired immune status is not the only unfavorable factor in these patients. Tobacco consumption, oral hygiene, genetic factors, previous history of periodontal disease are the main factors determining the status of periodontium [82]. It should be noted the strong correlation observed between smoking and attachment loss in HIV infected patients [83]

Impact of alcohol on periodontal diseases

Alcohol consumption is associated with the loss of attachment and increased severity of periodontal diseases [37,84]. It, along with smoking, is a major risk factor for deterioration of the oral health of individual [85]. In the future, there is a need of conduction of detailed studies on the role of alcohol as a factor for the development of periodontitis. It should be established whether there is a correlation between the type of alcohol (hard liquor, beer, wine), frequency of consumption, duration of use and the frequency and severity of periodontal diseases [36].

Impact of some systemic administered drugs on periodontal diseases

Calcium antagonists (especially nifedipine as a cheaper option) is widely used for the treatment of stenocardia, hypertension, heart rhythm disorders. This class of drugs produce gingival hyperplasia [18,86-89]. Nifedipine is associated most often with this complication. Between 10 and 20% of patients taking this medicine develop hyperplasia [87]. It is the result of the accumulation of a basic substance produced by activated fibroblasts. The authors are on the opposite opinion on whether Verapamil (another calcium antagonist), although similar in structure with Nifedipine, causes such a side reaction [86]. Some associate it with the induced gingival hyperplasia, together with the analogues Diltiazem, Nitrendipine, Felodipine [87]. Cyclosporin A is a potent immunosuppressant. It is used in tissue transplants. For the first time, in 1983 it was reported to cause gingival hyperplasia [86]. It is often used in combination with calcium blockers therefore it is difficult to determine the frequency of appearance of this complication. In 1995 Dzhemileva reported this type of hyperplasia [18]. Phenytoin, used to treat epilepsy, is another drug which use is associated with expansion of the gingiva [20,21,86,87]. Anticonvulsants such as Mephenitoin, Ethotoin, Phenobarbital, are often associated with gingival hyperplasia [87]. The modern society increasingly faces the problem of drug addicted patients. The different drugs act differently on the teeth and tissues in the oral cavity. The clinical picture includes rampantly ongoing caries, mucosal lesions, periodontal problems - refractory gingivitis and periodontitis. In Plovdiv in 2008 started the "Oral health in drug-addicted patients". Its purpose is to examine and classify the oral pathology in this type of patients. It was found that clinically diagnosed periodontal disease have 56% of the surveyed persons [90]. Prolonged smoking of marijuana also leads to alveolar bone loss [91].

Impact of occupational hazards on periodontal diseases

When working in hostile environment greater frequency and severity of periodontal diseases has been proved related to the presence of chemical, physical, biological agents [18]. In Plovdiv a study was conducted by FDM-Plovdiv, Department of Periodontology, in the connection with the prevalence of periodontal diseases among people working in an environment with chemical and physical hazards. It covers 319 workers at KCM-Plovdiv. Determined was the distribution of periodontal pathogens among workers in zinc production 100%, while in the leaden production 99.01% [92].

1.4. Systemic risk indicators

Impact of stress on periodontal diseases

Stress passing to distress is one of the systemic risk indicators for the development of periodontal disease [6,18,93,94]. Communication on the possible link between stress and this group of diseases appeared 50 years ago [93]. Subsequently, its effect on periodontal tissues has been studied in numerous experiments with humans and animals. The most pronounced is this relation in the acute necrotizing ulcerative gingivitis [18]. It is not possible in studies stress to be isolated and examined as an independent factor. In the stressed patients poor oral hygiene is often observed. Following the administration of specific drugs they develop xerostomia. Smoking habit is common habit with them [94]. In 1996 Moos conducted a study case - control (71 cases and 71 controls) and found that the risk of chronic periodontitis is three times higher in the studied stressed persons [93]. As reasons for stress he explores social factors - work, finances, family life. He unequivocally demonstrated the relation stress, depression, periodontitis. In 1998 - 1999 Genco performed a study involving 1426 people aged 24 to 74 and found high levels of cortisol in persons with severe periodontitis [95]. In 2000 - 2001 Deinzer examined students who are about to go to a hard exam and found that the study group has reduced oral hygiene and as a consequence develops gingivitis [96]. Stress causes disorder in homeostasis between microflora and defensive strength of the organism (Genco 1992, Ainamo 1996, Seymour 1996). It activates the autonomic nervous system to cause secretion of adrenaline and noradrenaline, which in their turn activate proteases and prostaglandins increasing the periodontal destruction [94]. A third group of authors explain the effect of stress with the adaptation syndrome of Selye [18,93]. When considering the impact of stress on periodontal diseases, it should be borne in mind that its role is limited. Stress is a potential risk factor, but not a major one. The successful treatment of necrotizing ulcerative gingivitis depends on the control of dental plaque, despite of the presence of stressful situations, smoking or diseases [93].

Impact of diet on the periodontal diseases

It is well known that diet can affect the immune system of the individual and the maintenance of tissue homeostasis. The inadequate nutrition itself does not cause periodontal inflammation, but the unbalanced diet leads to reduced resistance and inadequate reaction of the body against the infection [18]. Vitamin C affects the collagen synthesis. Scurvy or prolonged deficiency of this vitamin is characterized by severe periodontal changes [6,97]. The deficiency of vitamin D leads to osteomalacia in adults. This condition can cause destruction of the periodontal ligament and alveolar bone resorption [6,97]. Common in modern society is the state associated with low levels of calcium in the organism. Low calcium levels increase the risk of periodontitis especially among women over 30 and men over 60 [6]. Not surprisingly, osteoporosis and osteopenia in women in menopause are considered potential risk factors for periodontal pathogens [6]. Severe protein deficiency (kwashiorkor) or the generally expressed weakening (marasmus) are associated with increased gingival inflammation and bone loss. These changes are due to cell abnormalities - mediated, humoral or inflammatory responses in the presence of plaque-related disease [97]. Nowadays in developed countries such severe states of malnutrition is not observed [6]. However, there is an alternative problem - obesity, recognized as a risk factor for many chronic diseases - high blood pressure, diabetes and others. Obesity is also a systemic risk indicator for the occurence of periodontitis [6]. Studies in Japan and the USA discovered that people with high levels of fats in their body are more likely to develop periodontal disease if the factors of age, sex, health, etc. are eliminated [98-102]. It has been found that the frequency of feeding has an effect on the accumulation of dental plaque and a subsequent periodontal disease [97]. A study of Japanese scientists among 2,000 employees working in the chemical industry, showed that the probability of teeth loss has statistical significance in terms of the number of meals per day, inclusion of vegetables in the menu, the regularity of food intake, type of food [5]. The increased amount of fibers in food reduces the development of periodontitis due to a long chewing, leading to better self-cleaning of the teeth and reduction of plaque accumulation [6,97]. Adults may be prone to nutritional deficiencies as a result of edentulism, decreased salivation, impaired taste sensations, disorders such as Parkinson's disease and Alzheimer's disease [103]. A study from 1994 held in the USA covering a period of 10 years, did not establish an increased trend for tooth loss among adults compared with younger individuals [104,105].

Own study

In Bulgaria, data on the epidemiology of periodontal infection are scarce and there is no periodontitis register. The limited available data on periodontitis risk factors in Bulgaria, as well as the controversy in different authors' opinion, prompted the present study.

The present work was aimed at assessment of risk and analysis of risk factors for development of periodontitis in the studied patient population.

Patients and Methods
Patients

From November 2010 to February 2011, a study was conducted to assess the quality of life in 228 patients with chronic periodontitis. Participants were randomly selected from outpatients at the Department of Periodontology, Faculty of Dentistry, Medical University of Plovdiv (Bulgaria) and from various dentist surgeries in Plovdiv. All of them had sought treatment in the Department and the dentist surgeries.

Within the frame of the above-mentioned research, a pilot case-control study was conducted, including 80 patients (20 cases and 60 controls). It aimed to assess the risk of chronic periodontitis in the selected patients. The minimum sample size of patients was determined based on power analysis for sample size calculation. Age under 20 years was an exclusion criterion. The mean age of the participants was 31.33 ± 9.38 for the control group and 33.00 ± 11.52 for the case group.

Clinical method used for selecting the cases and controls

The periodontal health status was measured using The Community Periodontal Index (CPI) recommended by the World Health Organization (WHO) as a standard epidemiological examination method for periodontal disease, with dental mirror and WHO periodontal probe. Periodontitis was diagnosed based on the presence of clinically significant inflammation, peridontal osseous pockets and bone destruction. Thus, we selected 60 controls (randomly selected patients without periodontitis who had visited the dentist surgeries for other reasons) and 20 cases out of the 228 patients included in the primary survey. The cases included patients with chronic periodontitis who were matched to the controls, according to the most important socio-demographic parameters: sex, age, education. The aim was to eliminate the impact of obscuring factors. The case/control ratio was 1:3[106].

Sociological method

A direct, individual interview was performed with the participants from the cases and the control group. From the basic interview questionnaire (developed to assess the quality of life of the 228 patients with chronic periodontitis), only the sections related to risk factors assessment were used. The relevant sections were: socio-demographic characteristics of the patients cohort and presence of common risk factors prior to the development of periodontitis: smoking, alcohol abuse, stress, diabetes, vegetarian diet, fresh vegetable and fruit consumption, medication use, presence of hazards in the professional environment, level of oral hygiene, tooth clenching and grinding, regular calculus removal procedures, presence of overlapping and crooked teeth, regularity of dental examinations.

Statistical assessment

Descriptive statistics was used: analysis of variance, alternative analysis and non-parametric analysis (Fisher's exact test, t-test, Pearson criterion). Multiple logistic regressions were applied to evaluate the association between the variables (Backward Conditional procedure). Statistical significance was assumed at $P \leq 0.05$. SPSS ver.13.0 was applied for data processing.

In the process of data analysis, the categorical variables were recoded into dichotomous variables. The dependent variable was given two values: healthy subjects were assigned a value of "1" and patients were assigned a value of "0". Independent variables were coded in a similar manner. For instance, the independent variable smoking was assigned two values: negative response was coded as "1", meaning absence of periodontitis, and all positive responses were coded as "0". Only the variable regular fruit and vegetable consumption was coded in the reverse manner: regular consumption (positive response) was coded as "1" and negative response was coded as "0".

Results and Discussion

No statistically significant difference was observed in the socio-demographic parameters between cases and controls. The percentages according to sex, age and education are presented in **Table 1**.

Table 1. Socio-demographic characteristics of cases and controls.

Characteristics	Controls		Cases		Criterion	p
	n	%	n	%		
Education						
Secondary	34	56.67	10	50.00	$\chi^2 = 2.400$	0.493
High	26	43.33	10	50.00		
Total	60	100.00	20	100.00		
Age					$t = 0.420$	0.518
Mean age ± SD	31.33±9.38		33.00±11.52			
Sex						
Male	26	43.33	9	45.00	$\chi^2 = 0.017$	0.896
Female	34	56.67	11	55.00		
Total	60	100.00	20	100.00		

Most people in the studied sample were young adults: the mean age of controls was (31.33 ± 9.38) years, the mean age of cases was (33.00 ± 11.52) years. The number of females was slightly higher than that of males: the former were 56.67% of the patients in the control group and 55% in the cases group. The control group was comprised mostly of patients with secondary education (56.67%). In the cases group, the percentage of patients with higher education was equal to that of patients with secondary education.

In order to determine the strength of predictor variables for development of chronic periodontitis in the studied contingent, the effect size of each variable was investigated separately. Non-parametric analysis (Fisher's test) was used. The odds ratio (*OR*) and the 95% confidence interval (CI) for each of the 12 variables was calculated.

Table 2. Strength of predictor variables in the studied sample.

Variable	Controls n	Controls %	Cases n	Cases %	P	OR	95% CI
Smoking	28	46.67	9	45.00	0.35	1.39	0.50÷3.86
Alcohol use	34	56.67	8	40.00	0.15	0.51	0.18÷1.43
Hazards	3	5.00	1	5.00	0.08	0.19	0.02÷1.56
Stress	45	75.00	12	60.00	0.00	33.00	8.43÷129.19
Vegetarian diet	13	21.67	1	5.00	0.16	3.35	0.62÷18.16
Diet (lack of fresh fruit and vegetables in the daily menu)	10	16.67	4	20.00	0.48	0.80	0.22÷2.90
Oral hygiene (teeth brushing less than once daily)	7	11.67	5	25.00	0.22	0.29	0.03÷2.51
Calculus removal (none)	9	15.00	14	70.00	0.00	13.22	4.02÷43.47
Teeth clenching and grinding	10	16.67	7	35.00	0.08	2.69	0.85÷8.43
Crooked and overlapping teeth	12	20.00	15	75.00	0.00	12.00	3.63÷39.58
Diabetes	4	6.67	17	85.00	0.00	79.33	16.14÷389.92
Dentist practices visits (no visits or less than one visit annually)	14	23.33	18	90.00	0.00	0.03	0.01÷0.16

The statistical analysis (**Table 2**) showed that the following variables were statistically non-significant ($P > 0.05$) and they were excluded: smoking ($P = 0.349$), alcohol use ($P = 0.151$), vegetarian diet ($P = 0.162$), diet (lack of fresh fruit and vegetables in the daily menu) ($P = 0.485$), occupational hazards ($P = 0.080$), oral hygiene ($P = 0.225$), tooth clenching and grinding ($P = 0.081$). The significant variables ($P<0.05$) included: diabetes, stress, crooked and overlapping teeth, dentist practices visits and calculus removal.

Multiple logistic regressions (Backward Conditional procedure) were used to assess the combined impact of the selected significant variables (via one-factor analysis).

Table 3. Multifactor regression model of the predictor variables in the studied sample.

Variable	B (regression coefficient)	SE (standard deviation)	p
Diabetes	4.195	1.222	0.001
Crooked and overlapping teeth	3.022	1.118	0.010
Stress	2.882	1.236	0.014
Const.	-5.270	1.302	0.000

Following the multiple regression construct, three significant predictor variables were selected in the final equation: diabetes, stress, crooked and overlapping teeth. These factors showed the strongest relative weight in the studied cohort. The variable calculus removal is not present in the final equation ($P = 0.800$).

Based on the accumulated empirical data, a logistic model was constructed to assess the risk of periodontitis development. It incorporates the three selected variables: diabetes, stress, crooked and overlapping teeth. The model was shown to have a 93.80% predictive value ($\chi^2 = 63.91$; $P = 0.001$). Diabetes had the strongest predictive value (highest regression coefficient).

$$P = \frac{1}{1+e^{-(5.2+4.19(diabetes)+3.02(crooked\ and\ overlapping\ teeth)+2.88(stress))}} \qquad (0)$$

The selected predictor variables for development of periodontitis (**Table 2**) have been studied in a number of other research works[55-57,84,85,93-95]. None of the 80 interviewed patients in the case-control study indicated the use of therapeutic agents such as Verapamil, Nifedipin, Diltiazem, hydantoin medication, Cyclosporin A. For this reason, medication use (which has been studied as a factor by other authors) could not be investigated in our study. In the available reports, there is data that the above-mentioned therapeutic agents are related to the development of periodontitis [86,87]. In our study, only diabetes – as a systemic disorder – was incorporated in the statistical modeling, as none of the interviewed patients had indicated suffering from other genetic or immune-deficient disorders.

Interestingly, in the studied population, smoking was not selected as a risk factor for development of periodontitis. On the other hand, a number of other researchers have indicated cigarette use as one of the most important predictors for periodontitis [35-38]. Unlike their results, in the cohort studied by us, no statistically significant difference was established between the percentages of smokers in the control and the cases group: 46.66% ± 6.44% smokers in the cases group and 45.00% ± 11.12% in the control group. Our results indicated that in the studied population, smoking was not a significant factor for development of periodontitis ($P = 0.908$). This is likely due to the fact that our cohort was comprised mostly of young adults: 82.50% ± 4.24% of the patients belonged to the 20–39 age group. It seems that in these patients the duration of tobacco use was not long enough to induce a harmful effect on the periodontal tissues.

Similar results were obtained when the effect of alcohol use was studied. There was a statistically non-significant difference ($P = 0.247$) between the cases (56.67% ± 6.40%) and the controls (35.00% ± 10.66%). Therefore, alcohol did not prove to be a significant risk factor in our cohort. In similar cases, most authors recommend a more detailed investigation of the role of alcohol use in the pathogenesis of periodontitis. They focus on the correlation between frequency and severity of periodontitis and the frequency of alcohol consumption, the duration of alcohol consumption and the type of alcohol use (hard drinks versus beer and wine) [84,85]. Nonetheless, our study documents the negative trend typical of the Bulgarian society at present for a wider spread of two harmful habits, smoking and alcohol use.

The microorganisms in the tooth plaque are considered the major etiological factor inducing the pathological changes in the periodontal tissues [10-13]. The magnitude of plaque accumulations are largely dependent on the level of oral hygiene. Most patients in the studied group maintained good oral hygiene, only one person in each group indicated that they had never brushed his/her teeth ($P = 0.69$): in the control group (1.67% ± 1.65%) and in the cases group (5.00% ± 4.87%). Thus, poor level of oral hygiene was not proven a risk factor for periodontitis in the studied cohort.

Most Bulgarians share a traditional diet rich in meat and meat products. The current western trends for vegetarian diet are not yet widely spread in the Bulgarian society. Only five patients declared that they are vegetarians. Therefore, we could not establish a correlation between periodontitis development and vegetarian diet ($P = 0.162$). Similarly, no correlation was established between periodontitis and low consumption of fresh vegetables and fruit ($P = 0.485$).

In people exposed to occupational hazards (presence of chemical, physical and biological agents in the work environment), there is a higher frequency and severity of periodontal diseases [18]. A study with participants exposed to chemical and physical hazards in the city of Plovdiv (Bulgaria), reported the following incidence of periodontal diseases: 100% in zinc plant workers, versus 99.01% in lead production workers [92]. In our study, the percentage of patients with a history of exposure to professional hazard, was very low: 5.00% ± 2.81% in the control group and 5.00% ± 4.87% in the cases group. Therefore, in the studied cohort, exposure to professional hazards was not a significant predictor of periodontal disease ($P = 0.080$) most probably due to the small number of patients with such history that fell in the selected sample.

Based on Fisher's exact test, dentist practices visits were selected as a significant predictor of periodontitis. The calculated $OR < 1$ indicates that dental surgeon visits are not a risk factor, but have a protective effect against periodontitis in the studied contingent. Therefore, dentist practices examinations could aid the prophylaxis of periodontal diseases.

Periodontitis is a disease of multi-factor etiology and requires investigation of the complex effect of the risk factors. Logistic regression analysis can be applied to analyze the effect size and to determine the independent predictors for the development of periodontitis. The results from the regression analysis showed that three independent predictors of periodontitis can be selected: diabetes, stress and crooked and overlapping teeth (**Table 3**). Diabetes as a risk factor had the highest regression coefficient (B); thus, it had the strongest effect on the development of periodontitis. Similarly, other authors also document that periodontal disease is more frequent and severe in diabetic patients [55-57]. The second highest regression coefficient, after diabetes, was that of crooked and overlapping teeth. Stress was ranked third. Calculus removal, as a risk factor, was not present in the final equation ($P = 0.800$). Based on these findings, and the important role of diabetes as a risk factor, we recommend a closer cooperation between dental practitioners, endocrinologists and general practitioners, aimed at prevention, early detection and diagnosis of periodontal diseases.

Based on the three predictor variables with the strongest effect in the studied sample, a model of risk assessment was constructed. This model determined the least number of predictors (risk factors) that have the strongest predictor value in the development of periodontitis. The model was shown to have 93.80% predictive significance ($\chi^2 = 63.91$; $P = 0.001$)(**Fig.1**).

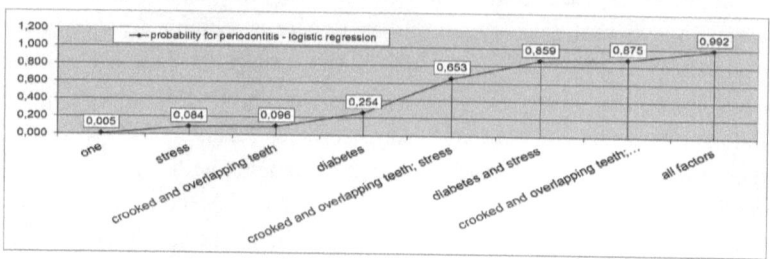

Figura 1. Model for assessing the risk of developing chronic periodontitis

This construct allows the dentists to undertake an adequate prophylactic approach in patients who have a history of risk factors for peridontitis, e.g. diabetes, crooked and overlapping teeth and stress.

A limitation of this pilot study is the small number of participants. Further investigation of the risk factors would need a more representative sample of patients. Future research should also include patients from various age groups, as mostly young adults were included in this study. This would allow estimating the effect of factors such as smoking and alcohol use.

Taken together, our results support the general understanding that integrated preventive strategies based on the common risk factors approach, are recommended for public health practice [107]. The national health authorities should ensure, therefore, that prevention of periodontal diseases is made an integral part of the prevention of diabetes and other chronic diseases, as well as of health promotion [107,108].

Conclusions

Our study included patients who reported exposure to some of the common risk factors for the development of periodontitis: diabetes, stress, crooked and overlapping teeth, poor oral hygiene, tobacco use, excessive alcohol consumption. The obtained results provided confirmatory evidence for the presence of risk factors for peridontitis. In our contingent, diabetes had a strongest predictive value in the development of the disease. Based on these findings, we recommend a closer cooperation between dental practitioners, endocrinologists and general practitioners, aimed at prevention, early detection and diagnosis of periodontal diseases. In order to investigate the impact of all factors for periodontitis described in the available literature, a larger number of patients of various age groups are needed.

Quality of Life

Quality of life is a multi-aspect concept concerning three main areas of an individual's life - physical, psychological and its social functioning.

In modern dentistry the issue of the impact of oral health on quality of life [109] comes to the fore, which requires the implementation of socio-biopsychological approach to the patient. There is evidence that oral health affects not only the physical condition of the individual, but also his/her social and psychological well-being. The interest in the concept of quality of life has increased in recent years. More than 1,000 new articles on this topic are indexed each year in the information network [110]. In a survey conducted in Medline, Dr. Mariko Naito found that the number of these articles between 2000 and 2004 was three times higher than in the period 1995-1999 [111]. The author and his team examined 1,726 articles which theme is the oral health related to the quality of life. Of them they chose five articles on the basis of their literary review, as in four significant correlation is accounted between oral diseases and quality of life. Problems with temporomandibular joint, dissatisfaction with the kind of teeth, complaints of dry mouth, were reported as the main causes of reduced quality of life of patients. The understanding of "quality of life" is purely subjective. The term includes the satisfaction of the human in life and the objective evaluation of his/her qualities and skills [112]. It includes the immeasurable in economic indicators subjective dynamic variable assessment of personal wealth and value of one's life [113]. According to Allison, this concept is not constant, but it undergoes changes over time [114]. This is the happiness which the individual experiences from health, marriage, financial state, self-confidence, creativity and others [115]. In 1995 WHOQOL Group defined quality of life as personal perception by the individual on his/her position in life in the context of cultural values that he/she professes, goals that he/she sets and expectations that he/she has [116]. The healthy person is free from restrictions, aches and pains. He is able to integrate in his/her social environment and feels part of the reality [113]. Given that the oral health is part of the overall health, then it definitely affects the quality of life.

Recently, supported is the view that quality of life related to health of the individual can be interpreted but not measured. In most cases, people define as good their quality of life when their biological and social functions are satisfied. Allen et al. have found that there is no correlation between the number of missing teeth and the quality of life of patients as interfering are other factors such as education, culture, income, lifestyle, food culture [117,118]. The lack of consensus in the medical literature regarding the definition of quality of life leads to the conclusion that the concept makes sense primarily on a personal level. In this regard, the health promotion center at the University of Toronto has developed a definition of quality of life that accepts this position and is consistent with the health promotion theory. It reads: "Quality of life refers to the degree to which a person enjoys the important opportunities in life" [119]. The definition can be simplified to answer the question: "How good is life for you?". This definition respects one of the basic ethical principles in medicine for protection of the autonomy and dignity of the individual.

Quality of life and oral health

The relation between quality of life and oral health is a dynamic concept. It includes concepts belonging to psychology, public health and medicine, as well as to improvement of the quality of life, which is the ultimate goal of any therapeutic effect [120]. This concept refers to the way the doctor treats the patient as a whole by coordinating dental health services with social and personal life of the patient. Oral health related to the quality of life is defined as assessment, both from the individual and from medical point of view, of the way in which these factors affect human well-being: functional, psychological (in terms of type and self-esteem of the person), social (interaction and perception), as well as pain and discomfort [121]. These groups of factors vary depending on individual, situation and impact on the environment [122].

In a study of oral health related to the quality of life studied were all the aspects of human life and the state of well-being as a consequence of all levels of medical care [117,122]. According to Reisine there is a need for a holistic approach in the study of social and psychological effects caused by oral diseases [123]. This is necessitated by the fact that the examination of these aspects on an individual level can affect the treatment decisions. Moreover, the quality of life depending on the oral health can become part and can determine the social policy of the country. In this regard, in the USA a study on the social impact of acute and chronic oral diseases was conducted by the National Health Survey. This influence is compared with the impact of such diseases as heart attack and neoplasms [123]. Thus the study of the relation between oral health and quality of life can be used not only as a tool for training of doctors, researchers and teachers, but also for health education of the public [124].

The assessment of the relationship between quality of life and oral health is included in the health policy of the developed countries. Main objective of the

Ministry of Health of the USA for 2010 is: "Increasing life expectancy and improving quality of life". The Secretary of Health, Donna D. Shalala, said in 2000 that: "The problems of dental health can generate useless pain and suffering, causing devastating complications. They lead to financial and social costs, which significantly worsen the quality of life and affect the American society "[125].

From the above facts it is obvious that the concept of "oral health related to the quality of life" includes new perspectives and emphasizes the transition from biomedical approach for health care which main objective is the treatment of the disease, to a new modern approach personality-centered medicine. The biopsychosocial model presented draws attention to all the problems of the patient, considered as a whole, based on the thesis: "There are no diseases, only sick people" [126].

Aspects of the impact of periodontitis on the quality of life

Oral diseases are progressive and have cumulative effect. Most of them are not fatal, but permanently damage the health as a result of the physical, psychological and social problems they create [127]. This requires a particular attention to these diseases, which should be based on their good knowledge and methods for their prevention. Periodontitis in its most common forms affects 5-15% of the population of industrial countries [6]. It leads to structural and functional changes in organs and tissues of the oral cavity, to recession of gums and formation of periodontal pockets [25]. The pockets may cause mobility of the teeth, gingival abscesses and tooth loss [25]. As one of the most common oral diseases periodontitis affects the quality of life, affecting its main aspects - physical, functional and psychological well-being, social activity of the individual [128-130]. It should be borne in mind that this influence is determined by the clinical form of periodontitis (mild, moderate, severe), respectively, by the depth of the periodontal pocket. Several studies show that stronger negative influence and burden of disability are seen in severe forms of periodontitis and depth of pockets greater than 4 mm. [131].

Periodontal diseases are one of the major causes for edentulism of the population globally - a problem with high social value [18,30]. Gerritsen A. and Finbarr P. carried out a systematic review and meta-analysis of the literature published from 1990 to 2009, on the relation between the number and the type of missing teeth and their impact on the oral health related to the quality of life. They prove that the burden of disability may be associated not only with the number but also with the type and distribution of the missing teeth. With the British and Greek population that association is relatively strong, but in other studies it depends on other factors [132]. According to a study in the last 50 years the process of edentulism has reduced by 10% per decade but the increase of the global population and the aging of the population compensate for this fact. The total edentulism is a chronic condition which contains all the components of disability [133]. The loss of teeth causes psychological trauma in the patient [30], which is just as significant as the loss of any other important organ of the body. The self-confidence of the individual is reduced, and the self-acceptance - distorted. The lack of teeth induces shame and attempt to hide the condition [134]. As with other events of a similar nature, the loss of teeth passes in five stages - denial, anger, depression, adaptation, adoption. Some individuals never overcome the state of depression from that loss. Such patients carry the stigma of the social discomfort that limits their contacts and isolates them, on the one hand, as a result of impaired aesthetics, and on the other hand, as a result of speech violation. Limiting the social activity of the individual can turn him/her into a social autist [129] and reduce his/her economic well-being [135]. According to a study carried out by Pearse and Thomson [136], oral diseases alter the social mobility of patients, i.e. their movement from one social group to another and the change of the social position is inextricably linked with the quality of life.

Periodontitis violates the aesthetic appearance of the individual, violating his/her self-acceptance, on the one hand, and, on the other hand, his/her perception by others.

Nowadays the aesthetic perfection has constantly increasing social importance, especially in Western societies, where the perfect smile and youthful appearance are prerequisites for social and commercial success [137]. Mouth and its area have a leading significance for the aesthetics of the face appearance [138]. It is believed that the beautiful people occupy a higher position in the social hierarchy, they find work easier, have higher incomes. It is natural that people, partially or completely toothless, will not be included in the imposed canons of beauty in the society. Because the face is a carrier of a rich aesthetic information which is the utmost significant factor for social interaction [138]. Namely social interaction and integration of the individual in the public life are one of the important indicators of the quality of life.

The communication of the individual in society is also hindered by speech disorders, which the lack of teeth causes. Human speech is main communicative means which on the biological terrain creates a new scar – the social one and it separates man from the rest of the living nature chain [139]. The relation between speech function and degree of edentulism has been demonstrated in several studies.

The first scientifically proven correlation between teeth and phonetics was documented by Oalley Coles in 1872 [139].

Periodontal diseases cause distortion of the functions in the mouth - chewing, swallowing, which affects the digestive system as a whole [140]. This problem occurs mainly in older patients where the risk for periodontal diseases and tooth loss is greater. The rehabilitation with prosthetic constructions recovers only 25% of the masticatory function [141]. A study conducted in England showed that totally toothless adult patients avoid certain types of foods - fruits and vegetables because they are difficult to chew [142]. Consequently, they have significantly lower plasma levels of ascorbic acid and retinol compared with levels in people with natural teeth. Therefore these patients are more susceptible to ocular and dermatological diseases.

There is a proven link between weight loss and chewing difficulties, causing the consumption of mashed food. Nutrition is one of the most easily achievable and lasting pleasures in life, even in people with poor health or disability. The different ways of preparing food offer opportunities for varied diet even in the absence of teeth. On the other hand, however, this type of diet is tasteless and unattractive and predisposes to anorexia and malnutrition, i.e. to decreased quality of life.

Recently the promotion of dental health reaches remarkable progress, but it must be borne in mind that the loss of natural teeth is associated largely with low socio - economic level and poor quality of life [143]. US studies show that 75% of people between 65-69 years of age are with natural teeth. It is believed that by 2030 the number of preserved natural teeth of adults will be doubled. This will increase the risk of periodontal diseases in this population group especially taking into consideration the aging of the population worldwide [25].

Several studies show that diverse pathology in the oral cavity definitely affects the quality of life of patients. This requires the introduction of tools to describe and quantify the impact of the oral health on the everyday life of the individual. These tools must also simultaneously consider the positive and negative aspects in the relation "oral health - quality of life" while at the same time associate this relation with demographic and socioeconomic parameters. With their help the priorities will be refocused, in particular of the dental health, and in a broader sense - the public health.

Tools for assessment of the impact of oral health on quality of life

In order to gather accurate data, needed for the planning of programs for prophylaxis and prevention of the diseases, as well as for a rational allocation of the health resources, it is not only important to correctly diagnose the disease but at the same time to measure the patient's personal perceptions of his/her health [144,145]. In modern literature messages to create different instruments (usually scales) in this direction increasingly find place.

In their own studies, Slade and Spencer prove that the instruments for measurement of oral health may be used to support the idea of the importance of oral health, especially when the objective is to provide public funding of the dental health care [146].

As number of studies relating to the definition of health as a concept and its relation to the quality of life grows, thus increases the need for the use of reliable tools to measure it. In the opinion of E. Scaret and A. Astrom they should be simultaneously effective, easily implement and easily manageable [147].

In modern dentistry generic instruments are used to measure the health status of the patient, and instruments based on the specifics of the disease. The benefits and limitations of both types of instruments are discussed below:

In the **first type** - generic tools for measuring health status – their psychometric properties that allow scales to be developed and comparisons be made between several populations with different problems, are considered as an advantage. These scales are not sensitive to the result of the dental care and respond poorly to changes in the properties [148].

The second type - instruments based on the specifics of the disease, have an advantage over the generic, as they are more likely to reflect even the slight changes in the specific properties and thus react more accurately. These methods are also sometimes not relevant in assessing the dental health, so Bowling offers them to be used in combination with the generic instruments [149]. Thus the first type can define the key areas in determining the quality of life of patients, and the second will improve the results of the study of various changes before and after treatment. Below are some of the specific instruments for measuring the health status, in the order of their creation.

AUTHOR	NAME OF INSTRUMENT
Cushinng et al. 1986	Social Impacts of Dental Disease
Atchison and Dolan 1990	Geriatric Oral Health Assessment Index
Strauss and Hunt 1993	Dental Impact Profile
Slade and Spencer 1994	Oral Health Impact Profile
Locker and Miler 1994	Subjective Oral Health Status Indicators
Leao and Sheiman 1996	Dental Impact on Daily Living
Adulyanon and Sheiman 1997	Oral Impacts on Daily Performances
McGrant and Bedi 2000	OH - QoL UK

However, the instruments for measurement of oral health-related quality of life (OHRQoL), are not widely used in dentistry. The need for a method based on how the patient himself/herself perceives his/her oral health has been recognized for the first time by Cohen and Jago. They point out that so far there are no data related to the psycho-social impact of the oral health problems [150]. In response to their findings, other scientists, as Reisine, start using social indicators such as job loss due to dental problems, to describe the social impact of oral diseases [151].

Reisine initially used the Sickness Impact Profile (SIP) tool to measure the outcome of the dental care [152]. This scale has also been validated by Bergner and his colleagues, and has long been widely used [153,154]. But this tool is a generic measure of the health status and can not be attributed to all oral health problems.

Similar is the opinion of Locker, who indicates that the scale measures the effects of acute and chronic diseases, but can not measure the consequences of the loss of teeth. The author states that in order to assess the health outcomes at the individual level, it is necessary to develop a tool based on individual perceptions of the patients [155].

Another method used to assess the specific problems of oral diseases is the General Oral Health Assessment Index (GOHAI) [156]. It has scales which provide an index of the impact of oral disorders related to the quality of life. It is calculated by giving an overall score indicating the degree of impact of each of the 12 groups of functional and psychosocial consequences. GOHAI contains 12 questions (e.g., "How often do you feel embarrassed to eat in front of other people, because of problems with your teeth or dentures?") with the following possible answers (never = 0, rarely

= 1, sometimes = 2, often = 3; very often = 4; always = 5). The coded responses are aggregated for all 12 questions in order to give an overall score of 0 to 60. A similar approach is used by Locker and Miller in the development of Subjective Oral Health Status Indicators [157].

Advantage of the innovative model of Wolinsky and Wolinsky is that it is focused on three main aspects of the health status of the individual: physical, social and psychological [158]. The physical aspect is measured in terms of the physician and reflects the traditional medical model. The social aspect is measured in terms of the public regarding the objectives and the implementation of the roles of the individual and the psychological is measured on a personal level and reflects the sense of satisfaction and happiness.

These three aspects are used in the construction of the instrument Social Impact of Dental Diseases (SIDD), developed in the early 1980s [159]. It is one of the first socio-dental indicators, a response of the expressed dissatisfaction with the conventional scales of health assessment that fail to measure the impact of diseases and thus the outcome of the health services on the well-being of the people [159]. The development of the indicator was influenced by the debate about what constitutes the quality of life. The concept is present in the formulation of the public health policy and the setting of the priorities in the allocation of the health resources [160]. With this tool, based on interviews for measurement of the social and psychological impact of dental diseases, five categories of influence are outlined: dietary restrictions, in communication, pain, discomfort, aesthetic frustration. Pain and discomfort are separated as categories. The end result is obtained by the sum of the results of several categories. Result 1 is given to the category in which a positive response is given to all questions. Symptoms ""bad breath" and "taste" are excluded from the total result, because they are caused by various factors and are not necessarily associated with the teeth. Two final results are used - the one including (total score of 0- 5) and the other excluding discomfort (0- 4) [159].

OHIP-14 (Oral Health Impact Profile) was originally developed in Australia on the basis of the conceptual model for oral health and uses the international classification of disability of the WHO. The original instrument consists of 49 questions that were made redundant by Slade to 14 and this shortened version is much more convenient to use [161,162]. Its questions are divided into seven theoretical areas - functional disability, pain, psychological discomfort, physical disability, psychological disability, social disability, difficulties. Sample question is: "Have you ever had cases of difficulty eating because of problems with the teeth, mouth, dentures?". The following responses are used: 0 = never; 1 = almost never; 2 = occasionally; 3 = fairly often; 4 = very often. This instrument is considered to be the most complicated in the measurement of the impact of oral health [163]. It only takes into account the negative impact of oral health on the quality of life [164]. Its main advantage is that the results obtained from the evaluation of the patients for their condition, and are not detected by clinical methods by dentists. It can be used to identify groups of patients, priorities for the reception of dental care.

In the United Kingdom, Mc Grath et al. developed the tool Oral Health - Related Quality of Life (OHQuL-UK). It consists of 16 questions divided into four sections covering the social status of the patient, his/her psychological and physical condition and symptoms of the disease [165]. The version of Mc Grath accounts the positive and negative effects of oral health on the quality of life of the patients, which is an advantage over the use of OHIP-14.

OIDP (Oral Impact on Daily Performance) is another tool that tries to determine the relative frequency of the impact of oral health problems in the daily life and activities of the individual, namely in the following areas: nutrition and enjoyment of food, speech and clear pronunciation, dental hygiene, sleep and rest, smile and laugh, when the patient shows his teeth without shame, normal work and social activity, maintaining a normal emotional state, without showing irritability, delight of communication with the surrounding [166-168].

Possible answers range from 0 (in the past 6 months these activities were not affected) to 5 (every or almost every day were affected). Respondents were asked to evaluate the severity of the impact using a scale from 0 to 5. As an advantage of the tool can be specified the evaluation of the emotional nuances of the various functions. It has good validity, it is short, but at the same time it covers aspects such as pain and problems with chewing. In future it must be subjected to a long-term study in order to establish its sensitivity to changes after treatment and to be applied to populations of different ethnic groups and cultures.

The Dental Impact on Daily Living (DIDL) tool examines 36 elements grouped into five areas: comfort, appearance, pain, work and restriction diet [169]. The impact of each element is encoded with (+1) for a positive impact; (-1) for negative; (0) has no effect. Each area is assessed individually by dividing the total responses for each element in it by the maximum possible sum. This tool seeks to measure how each individual perceives his/her oral health i.e. how to measure the frequency and severity of oral problems affecting the quality of life of the patient. Further studies are needed in the future to demonstrate its sensitivity

The Dental Impact Profile scale is based on the concept that the state of the dentition can have a positive or negative aspect on the quality of life of the patient. Its advantages are that it allows for the consideration of cultural and ethnic differences and their impact on health. It is short and easy to use. It can be used in the area of marketing of health services and their promotion. A shortcoming of the tool may be the fact that the interviewer can suggest the respondent.

The problems associated with measuring and evaluating the quality of life in patients with oral diseases, have been developed recently in Bulgaria. In 2006 M. Bratoycheva developed her own scale for assessing the quality of life of patients with cancer of the oral cavity. It is a five-level scale and it accounts the violations in speech and nutritional functions and distortions in the appearance of the patient. The assessment is done by a dentist. Further, with the help of an interview the patient's view of social and psychological problems caused by the disease is examined.

The author is on the opinion that if the scale of assessment of the quality of life is implemented in the clinic of maxillofacial surgery, this will facilitate the social rehabilitation and management of health care [170].

Use of tools for oral health

Despite the application of a series of detailed and complex tools for measuring of the oral health, yet in practice their mass use has yet not been applied, the largest deficit is observed in tools based on perceptions of the patient on his/her oral health. These scales have been used mostly in descriptive studies of adults, which have found that the problems in oral health have a significant impact on functional and psychosocial well-being of the individuals [171-175]. In one of these studies Slade et al. examined the social impact of oral health in 6 groups of the population over the age of 65 with different economic and social status [172].

Sheiham et al. used OIDP in the UK and proved that the loss of teeth has a significant negative effect on the process of eating and speech [175]. Despite the development and use of scales with a solid theoretical basis, some issues remain unresolved, such as which tool exactly should be used in a particular case. It is still difficult to give an answer to this question because there are no scientific studies that clearly demonstrate the effectiveness of one or another method. There are not enough studies on the applicability of tools for assessing the impact of clinical intervention. Significant barrier to the use of these measures is the large number of elements that should be included for study. While the shorter versions are easier to apply, the reliability of their index may decrease the exclusion of certain elements. For example, the short version of OHIP contains 14 points obtained from 49 elements of OHIP-49, but it exhibits good validity and reliability. To assess the result of clinical procedures GOHAI tool is much easier and more convenient to use than OHIP, for instance. Almost all of the above scales are not developed as indices for evaluation, and therefore can not be used alone and applied in addition to the clinical methods.

Despite the complexity of the developed tools for measuring the oral health, they must find application in practice to make the connection between the professional assessment of the dentist about the need for treatment and the subjective evaluation of the patient. Thus the patient will identify himself/herself with the problem and his/her motivation for treatment will be increased. Clinicians should be encouraged to collect and interpret the data, and the international scientific community must develop a strategy for comparing them, taking into account that the effects of oral diseases vary between populations with different cultural backgrounds [176]. Health models endure continuous development, making it necessary to assess whether the existing tool for measuring the oral health are strong enough and effective or new ones should be developed.

Evaluation of the impact of chronic periodontitis on individual's Quality of life using a self-developed tool

A number of studies show that periodontitis influence the Quality of Life (QoL) of patients, affecting negatively the physical, functional and psychological well-being and social activity of individuals [3,4,5,6,7,8,9,10,11]. More severe stages of periodontitis associated with greater depth of periodontal pockets, mobility and displacement of teeth have a greater negative impact [2,4]. In this type of studies different already established tools for assessment of oral health-related quality of life such as OHIP, GOHAI, OIDP have been applied [5,6,10]. Although they have been widely used through the years and have proved their worth in evaluation, it is difficult to determine which of those tools is most effective.

In Bulgaria no studies have been conducted so far on the QoL of patients with periodontitis. This fact, as well as the negative trends in the oral health conditions of Bulgarians, gave occasion to the authors to develop their own scale for evaluating the impact of periodontitis on QoL.

Purpose

Aim of the present study was to administer the self-developed tool in order to evaluate the impact of chronic periodontitis on QoL among a sample of individuals.

Materials and methods

The research/ patients:

From November 2010 to February, 2011, a cross-sectional study was conducted to evaluate the impact of chronic periodontitis on QoL. The sample was a group of patients enrolled for care at the Department of Parodontology, Faculty of Dentistry, Plovdiv, Bulgaria and from various city dental surgeries. 228 patients were selected by convenience. The minimum sample size of patients was established based on power analysis for sample size calculation. Age < 20 years was an exclusion criterion. Patients were between 20-80 years of age, from both genders. All of the patients were informed about the purpose of the research and gave their agreement to participate. All participants were clinically diagnosed with chronic periodontitis. The diagnosis of chronic periodontitis was established through records of periodontal parameters (clinical attachment level and probing depth) and periapical radiographs. The degree of chronic periodontitis is classified as mild periodontitis, in wich there is attachment loss of 1-2 mm; moderate periodontitis, when the attachment loss is 3 to 4 mm; and severe periodontitis, when the attachment loss is 5 mm or more. Direct, individual interviews were performed with all 228 patients. **Pilot study**

A pilot research was conducted for the validation of face and content validity of the scale. The internal and external consistency of the scale was tested. Thirty patients were interviewed *(n=30)*, using a pilot version of the tool. The minimum sample size of 30 people has been established based on a power analysis. After three months the same patients were interviewed again with the same questionnaire for the purpose of testing the stability of the scale and its reliability during the whole period of research.

Data gathering

A new original tool was designed and developed. The design phase of the scale included defining its content (writing of items) and construction of its format (type of the scale). The initial version contained 11 items:

Table 4. Questions in the initial version of the pilot research

1. Do you consider that the conditions of your gums/ teeth have an influence on your outlook;
2. Do you consider that the conditions of your gums/ teeth have an influence on your self-esteem;
3. Do you consider that the conditions of your gums/ teeth have an influence on your general health;
4. Do you consider that the conditions of your gums/ teeth have an influence your choice of food;
5. Do you consider that the conditions of your gums/ teeth might cause problems in chewing of harder food;
6. Do you consider that the conditions of your gums/ teeth might cause problems in swallowing;
7. Do you consider that the conditions of your gums/ teeth might cause speaking difficulties
8. Do you consider that the conditions of your gums/ teeth have an influence on your family life;
9. Do you consider that the conditions of your gums/ teeth have an influence on professional life;
10. Do you consider that the conditions of your gums/ teeth have an influence on your social contacts;
11. Have you ever received a negative comments from your friends and relatives in regards to your gums/teeth;

Authors grouped the above 11 items into the following three subscales:

1. Choice of food/nutrition, chewing, swallowing, talking; (Do you consider that the conditions of your gums/ teeth: influence your choice of food; chewing of harder food; cause problems in swallowing, cause speaking difficulties)

2. Social relations, friends and family, professional life; (Do you consider that the conditions of your gums/ teeth: have an influence on your self-esteem; your outlook; family life; professional and social contacts. Have you ever received a negative comments from your friends and relatives in regards to your gums/teeth)

3. Overall health (Do you consider that the conditions of your gums/ teeth have an influence on your general health)

Coding of the answers: Answers to every question were coded in a five-degree ranked scale depending on the degree of their influence (incl. 0 points when the patient considered that the relevant answer did not have any influence):

1 p. - insignificant influence;
2 p. - weak influence;
3 p. - moderate influence;
4 p. - strong influence;
5 p.- extremely strong influence;

The points of all answers were summed up to give a total score which was used as a base for a comprehensive assessment of the impact of periodontitis on QoL. The maximum total score could reach up to 45 points. In case of gathered up to 11 points- periodontitis had an insignificant influence, up to 18 points-its impact on QoL was small, up to 27 points- moderate, up to 33 points - strong and over 34 points it was extremely hard. Overall rating (the sum of the points from the answers of all the questions) varied from 0 to 45 total score.

Statistical processing
The results were processed statistically with the help of SPSS Statistical Package for Social Science – version.13. First, the internal consistency was assessed with the coefficient of Cronbach (Cronbach's alpha). Second, the changing factors were researched using the coefficients of Pearson *(r)* and Spearman – Brown (r_{sb}). After wards in the research authors checked the reliability of the result by a performed test-retest analysis. The next step was to conduct an item analysis and to calculate the difficulty and discrimination power of all questions. Authors measured the difficulty as a proportion in which the average value refers to the maximum value, as the lowest level of response was coded with "0". The discrimination power was measured by the coefficient of linear correlation between the item rating and the overall unprocessed rating, from which the according item was excluded.

Results
Sample description
The study involved 228 patients distributed in three age groups (Table 2). The mean age of participants was 50.35±9.85. Male patients were 97 (42.54±3.27%) and the female - 131 (57.46±3.27%) **(Table 5)**.

Table 5. Characterization of the sample

Age group	Male		Female		Total	
	n	%	n	%	n	%
20-39 years	26	26,80	29	22,14	55	24,12
40- 59 years	50	51,55	71	54,20	121	53,07
Up 60 years	21	21,65	31	23,66	52	22,81
Total	97	100,00	131	100,00	228	100,00

The patients with mild periodontitis were 34.2%, with moderate chronic periodontitis were 24.6% and with severe chronic periodontitis were 41.2% (**Table 6**). When assessing the type of chronic periodontitis according to the demographic variables, a statistically significant difference was found with regard to age – 59% of those with severe chronic periodontitis were over 60 years old (**Table 6**).

Table 6. Assessment of the type of periodontitis according to age group

Age group	Patients with periodontitis							
	Mild		Moderate		Severe		Total	
	n	%	n	%	n	%	n	%
20-39 years	10	13	5	7,1	1	1	16	7
40- 59 years	64	82	32	10,7	38	40	134	58,8
> 60 years	4	5	19	14,3	55	59	78	34,2
Total number	78	100	56	100	94	100	228	100

Reliability and validity
After the conduction of the above explained pilot research among 30 diagnosed patients with chronic periodontitis the face and content validity of the instrument were confirmed. The Cronbach's alpha coefficient value in the initial version of the pilot research was equal to ($\alpha=0.882$), the Spearman - Brown coefficient- ($r_{sb}=0.998$). Its high value confirmed the reliability of the scale. After the statistical processing of the pilot version, two of the questions had to be excluded from the initial questionnaire (**Table 7**)

Table 7. Correlation coefficients between the items (initial version)

	Correlation coefficients between the items (initial version- 11 questions)										
Q	1	2	3	4	5	6	7	8	9	10	11
1	1										
2	0.869	1									
3	0.851	0.775	1								
4	0.445	0.487	0.513	1							
5	0.440	0.435	0.415	0.786	1						
6	0.273	0.288	0.273	0.495	0.564	1					
7	0.394	0.373	0.296	0.633	0.747	0.784	1				
8	0.459	0.542	0.359	0.459	0.271	0.153	0.323	1			
9	0.467	0.576	0.382	0.288	0.113	-0.112	0.121	0.780	1		
10	0.705	0.779	0.500	0.289	0.124	0.199	0.280	0.662	0.672	1	
11	0.252	0.306	0.098	0.327	0.373	0.031	0.428	0.396	0.368	0.249	1
Average value of the inter-item correlations											
R=0.425											

After the second processing of the rest nine questions, the received results were as follows: Coefficient of Cronbach was $\alpha=0.883$, the Coefficient of Spearman – Brown was $r_{sb}=0.998$, the value of the Average inter item correlation coefficient was $R=0.507$; the values for Difficulty of questions: $min = 0.287$, $max= 0.757$. Furthermore authors defined the Discrimination power values as follows: the lowest was (0.524) and the highest was (0.809)(**Table 8**).

Table 8. Difficulty and discrimination power of the 9 questions after the elimination

Difficulty and discrimination power of the 9 questions after the elimination (second version)									
Question N	1	2	3	4	5	7	8	9	10
Difficulty T_i	0.717	0.690	0.757	0.500	0.470	0.287	0.390	0.413	0.553
Discrimination power	0.765	0.809	0.662	0.667	0.552	0.524	0.665	0.564	0.656

Assessing the impact of parodontitis on individual's QoL using the self-developed tool

The evaluation of the impact of chronic periodontitis on QoL according to the overall sum of points for each patient and the degree of disease is presented in **Table 9**.

Table 9. Assessment of the influence of periodontitis on the QoL of patients in the sample based on the scale

Influence of periodontitis	Patients with periodontitis							
	Mild		Moderate		Severe		Total	
	n	%	n	%	n	%	n	%
Do not Influence	45	58	4	7,1	1	1	18	7,9
Influence incignificant	14	17,9	6	10,7	5	5	22	9,7
Small	10	12,8	8	14,3	10	11	60	26,3
Moderate	7	9	32	57	12	13	55	24
Strong	2	2,6	2	3,6	39	41	42	18,4
Extremalystrong	0	0	4	7,1	27	29	31	13,6
Total number	78	100	56	100	94	100	228	100

The results showed that severe chronic periodontitis had strong (41%) and extremely strong (29%) negative impact on QoL.

Through the study process the areas of periodontitis' influence with the highest impact on QoL have been researched (**Fig. 2**)

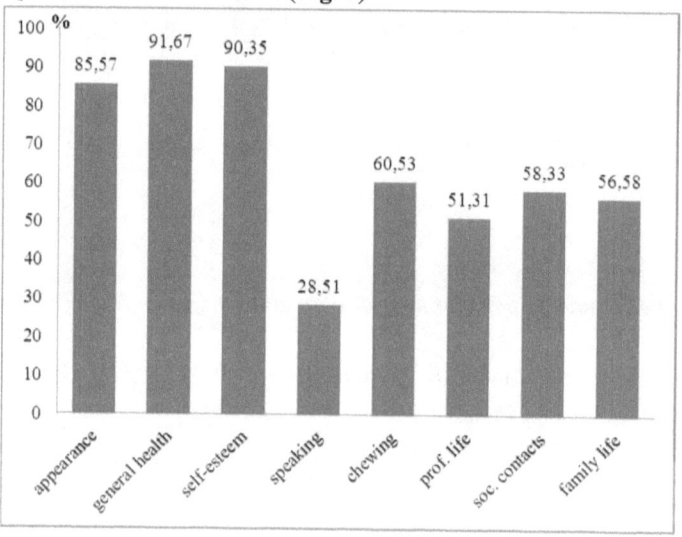

Figure 2. Areas of patients' QoL influenced by the chronic periodontitis.

The most prevalent domain was general health - 91.67% followed by self-esteem and appearance, least affected function was speaking - 28.51%.

Discussion

This study is the first research to use such an instrument in measuring oral health related QoL in Bulgaria. The scale is a precise, valid and a reliable disease specific instrument. The high value of the coefficient Cronbach's alpha in the present case equal to ($\alpha=0.882$) proved the reliability of the instrument. Two questions occurred to be problematic during the research of the internal consistency - the question of related to "swallowing problems" and to "negative comments by the closest friends and relatives". When calculating their correlation with the rest of the items (inter-item correlations), the result were extremely minimal values and even a negative value in one of the cases *(-0.112)*. In the present research the coefficients of the discrimination power were relatively equal and with high values (varied in the range of *0.405- 0.809*) with the exception of the above described two questions *(0.405)* and *(0.417)* where the lowest values were observed. The authors explained this with the fact that both questions are logically connected with already asked before questions. In the first case the chewing of harder food and the process of swallowing were in a close relation. In the other question the negative comments of the closest friends and relatives were directly related to family life and social contacts which patients had already commented. This was the logical ground on which these questions have been eliminated from the second statistical processing of data and thus the final version of the instrument consists of nine questions.

The present study include a greater number of women in the sample. This observation is a common finding in institutional samples that may be explained by cultural moorings that hinder the adoption of self-care practices in males.

The questions of the self-developed tool are formulated on the basis of literature analysis exploring various aspects of the periodontitis impact on QoL [109,110]. The evaluation of the periodontitis influence on the QoL of patients was done by summing the number of points that brings the answer to each of the nine questions. Higher points score means a stronger negative impact and thus deteriorated QoL. After calculating the total score points of each of the respondents, it was found that periodontitis had small or no effect on QoL only in 18% of cases, and in the remaining 82% it was established varying degrees of influence - strong and very strong at 32% respondents and moderate in 24%. The present study on the impact of chronic periodontitis on the QoL revealed that negative aspects were more prevalent among individuals with severe chronic periodontitis – 41% of patients with severe chronic periodontitis reported strong influence of disease and 29% extremely strong (**Table 9**).These results stated clearly that the QoL of most patients was worsened. The result coincided with the conclusions of other authors who also demonstrated the negative impact of periodontitis on QoL but using different (OHIP, OIDP) than the current self- developed instrument [110,164-166,177].

The literature review showed that among patients with periodontitis the functional limitations were leading- problems with chewing and swallowing [177]. Those authors reported that eating disorders usually occur in older patients [178-182]. In the current study the results were different. The physical aspect of the periodontitis influence had the most profound impact on researched contingent (appearance and general health) followed by the psychological discomfort - reduced self-esteem. The outcome can be explained by the dominance of women in the survey who are more conscious about those factors. Least affected function was speaking. Large share of the patients' sample had already recovered their orthopedic defects in tooth rows and therefore not reporting disturbance of speech function.

This present study exhibits some limitations such as the sample consisted of periodontally compromised patients who sought treatment in a specialized clinics, with no control group of healthy patients for the comparison of results and participantes in the study could have other oral cavity disease (tooth loss, caries, malocclusions) that may also have negative effects on quality of life.

Conclusions

The evaluation of QoL of patients with chronic periodontitis based on the developed tool shows that chronic periodontitis had an impact on quality of life and the most prevalent negative aspects were found in patients with severe chronic periodontitis. Most strongly affected areas are the appearance, self-esteem and overall health of individuals.

The scale can be successfully utilized in practice, which will help dentists to quickly and easily evaluate the QoL of patients with periodontitis.

Periodontitis is the second largest oral health problem, affecting 10-15% of the world's population, Taking these results into account, if dental practitioners are presented with the elaborated model for assessing the risk of developing chronic periodontitis, it will be possible, as early as upon taking the patient's history and in the presence of the factors of diabetes, stress, misshapen and overlapping teeth, to apply a more adequate prophylactic approach to periodontitis and the prevention of its development.

References

1. Palma P, Caetano P, Leite I. Impact of periodontal diseases on health related quality of life of users of the Brazilian Unified Health Systems. http://dx.doi.org/10.1155/2013/150357
2. Escudero Castano N, Perea Garcia M. Revision de la periodontitis chronica. Evulacion y su aplicasion clinica. *Av en Period* 2008; 20(1):27.
3. Fereira Lopes M, Gusmao E. The impact of chronic periodontitis on quality of life in brazilian subject. Acta Stomatol Croat 2009; 43 (2): 89-98.
4. Baelum V, Luan WM, Chen X et al. A 10-year study of the progression of destructive periodontal disease in adult and eldery Chinese. *J Periodontol 1997;* 68: 1033.
5. Loe H. Periodontal disease as we approach the year 2000. *J Periodontol* 1994; 65: 464-467.
6. Clerehugh V, Tugnait A, Genco R. Periodontology at a Glance. Wiley-Blackwell 2009.
7. Seymour G. Importance of the host response in the periodontium. *J Chn Periodontol* 1991; 18: 421-426.
8. Hart T, Shapira L, Van Dyke T. Neutrophil defects as risk factors for periodontal diseases. *J Periodontol* 1994; 65: 521-529.
9. Rioboo Crespo, Bascones A. Risk factors for periodontal disease: the genetics factors. *Av en Period* 2005; 17 (2):69-77.
10. Bascones Martinez A, Figuero Ruiz E. Las enfermedades periodontales como infections bacterianas. *Av Periodon Implantol* 2005; 17(3): 147-156.
11. Escribano M, Matesanz P. Pasado, presente y futuro de la microbiologia de la periodontitis. *Av in Periodoncia* 2005; 17 (2): 79- 87.
12. Offenbacher S. Periodontal diseases: pathogenesis. *Ann Periodontol* 1:821, 1996.
13. Zambon JJ. Periodontal diseases: microbial factors. *Ann Periodontol* 1:879, 1996.
14. VS Department of Commerce, Burean of the census: Census 2000 brief, 2001, http://www.census. Gov.
15. Schei O et al. Alveolar bone loss as related to oral hygiene and age. *J Periodontol* 1959; 30 (1): 7-16.

16. Sheiman A. Dental cleanliness and chronic periodontal disease. Studies of populations in Britain. *Brit Dent J* 1970; 129: 413.
17. Waerhaug J. Prevalence of parodontal disease in Ceylon. *Acta Odont Scand* 1967; 25: 205-209.
18. Djemileva T. Periodontal diseases. Acer Sofia, 1999.
19. Baelum V, Luan WM, Chen X et al. A 10-year study of the progression of destructive periodontal disease in adult and eldery Chinese. *J Periodontol 1997;* 68: 1033.
20. Douglas CW, Jette AM, Fox CH et al. Oral health status of the eldery in New England. *J Gerontol* 1993; 48 (2): 39-46.
21. Burt BA, Ekland SA. Dentistry, dental practice and the community, ed 4. Philadelphia: W.B. Sanders 1992; p. 339.
22. James D, Beck J, Samuel J et al. Epidemiology of gingival and periodontal diseases. In: Newman M, Takei H, Klokkevold P. Carranza "s clinical periodontology 2006. P. 125-126.
23. Abdellatif HM, Burt BA. An epidemiological investigation into the relative importance of age and oral hygiene status as determinants of periodontitis. *J Dent Res* 1987; 66: 13.
24. Burt BA. Periodontitis and aging : reviewing recent evidence. *J Am Dent Assoc* 1994, 125: 273.
25. Needleman I. Periodontal treatment for older adults. In: Newman M, Takei H, Klokkevold P. Carranza "s clinical periodontology 2006,p 93-98.
26. Clerehugh V, Lennon MA, Worthington HV. 5-years results of a longitudinale study of early periodontitis in 14 to 19 year old adolescents. *J Clin Periodontol* 17:702, 1990.
27. Page RC, Beck JD. Risk assessment for periodontal disease. *Int Dĕnt J* 1997; 47: 67.
28. Taylor W, Borgnakke W. Self- reported periodontal disease. Validation in an epidemiological survey. *J Periodonto* 2007; 78: 1407-1420.
29. Nevins M. Essential of Periodontal Treatment Planing for adult chronic periodontit. In: Nevins M, Melloning J. Perodontal therapy. Clinical Approaches and Evidence of Success. Quintessence Publishing Co, Inc. 1998,p. 20
30. Kiselova A, Krastev Z, Kolarov R. Oral medicine. Sofia 2009.
31. Niessen LC, Channcey HH. Geriatric dentistry: aging and oral health. St Louis 1991, Mosby.

32. Borrell LN, Crawford ND. Social disparities in periodontitis among US adults 1999-2004. *Community Dent Oral Epidemiol* 2008; 36: 383-391.
33. AIHW Dental Statistics and Research Unit. Research Report 9. Social determinants of Oral Health. *Am J Dent* 2004; 17: 307-309.
34. Novak JM, Novak KF. Smoking and periodontal disease. In: Newman M, Takei H, Klokkevold P. Carranza "s clinical periodontology 2006: 251-258.
35. Yoshida Y, Hatanaki Y, Imaki M. Tooth loss and lifestyle factors. *J of Physiological anthropology* 2001; 20(6) : 369-373.
36. Takashi H, Ojima M, Tanak K. Casual assessment of smoking and tooth loss. A systematic rewiew of observational studies. *BMC Oral Health* 2011; 11: 221.
37. Labriola A, Needleman I. systematic rewiew of the effect of smoking on nonsurgical periodontal therapy. *Periodontot 2000*; 2005; 37: 124-137.
38. Heasman L, Stacey F, Mc Gracken GI. The effect of smoking on periodontal treatment response: a review of clinical evidence. *J Clin Period* 2006; 33: 241-243.
39. Osorio Gonzales AY, Bascones Martinez A, Villarroel Dorego M. Salivary ph alterations in smoker patients with periodontal disease. *Av en Periodoncia* 2009; 21(2): 75-79.
40. Leyva Huerta ER. Actividad de la lactado deshidrogenosa en fluido crevicular gingival y saliva en fumadores con periodontitis chronica. *Av en Periodoncia* 2009; 21(2): 21-26.
41. Glick M. The effect of alcohol and tobacco habits on oral health. In: Di Annual World Dental Congress, 2-5 sept. 2010. Final Programme (Abstract Book) p.91.
42. Locker D, Leake JL. Risk indicators and risk markers for periodontal disease experience in older adults living independently in Ontario, Canada. *J Dent Res* 1992; 72 (1): 9-17.
43. Bergstrom J, Preber H. Tabacco use as a risk factors. *J Periodontot* 1994; 65: 545-560.
44. Position paper: Tabacco use and the periodontal patient. *J Periodontol* 1999; 70: 1419.
45. Papapanou PN. Risk assessment in the diagnosis and treatment of periodontal disease. *J Dent Educ* 1998; 62: 822.
46. Tonneti MS. Cigarette smoking and periodontal disease: etiology and management of disease. *Ann Periodontol* 1998; 3: 88.

47. Rider M. Tabacco use. In: Wilson T, Kornman K. The base of periodontology. Medical Pub. Sharov. Sofia 1999. p. 200-204.
48. Linden GJ, Mullally BH. Cigarette smoking and periodontal destruction in young adults. *J Periodontot* 1994; 65: 718-728.
49. Tomar SL, Asma S. Smoking attributable periodontitis in the US: findings from NHANES 3. *J Period* 2000; 71: 743.
50. Zambon JJ, Grossi SG, Machtei EE et al. Cigarette smoking increase the risk for subgingival infection with periodontal patogens. *J Period* 1996; 67: 1050.
51. Bennet RR, Read PC. Salivary Im A levels in normal subject, tobacco smokers, and patients with minor aphtous ulceration. *Oral Surg Oral Med Oral Pathol* 1982; 53:461-465.
52. Schenkein HA, Gunsolley JC, Koertge TE et al. Smoking and its effects on early – onset period. *J Am Dent Assoc* 1995;126: 1107.
53. Holm G. Smoking as an additional risk for tooth loss. *J Period* 1994; 65: 996.
54. Krall EA, Garvey AJ, Garcia RJ. Alveolar bone loss and tooth loss in male cigar and pipe smokers. *J Am Dent Assoc* 1999; 130: 57.
55. Rise T, Halmo U. Endocrine diseases. In: Wilson T, Kornman K. The base of periodontology. Medical Pub. Sharov. Sofia 1999. p. 210-212.
56. Genco R. Periodontal complication of diabetes. In : Di Annual World Dental Congress, 2-5 sept. 2010. Final Programme: p. 68 (Abstract Book).
57. Van Dyke T. Inflamation and diabetes. In: Di Annual World Dental Congress, 2-5 sept. 2010. Final Programme: p. 67 (Abstract Book).
58. Loe H. Periodontal disease: The sixt complication of diabetes mellitus. Diabetes care 1993; 16(1):329-34.
59. Tervonen T, Oliver RC. Long term control of diabetes mellitus and periodontitis. *J Clin Periodontol* 1993; 20: 431.
60. Westfelt E, Rylander H, Blohme G et al. The effect of periodontal therapy in diabetics; results after 5 years. *J Clin Period* 1996; 23: 92.
61. Oliver RC, Tervonen T. Diabetes: a risk factor for periodontitis in adults. *J Period* 1994; 65: 530.
62. Genco RJ, Lde H. The role of systematic conditions and disordes in periodontal disease. *Periodontology 2000*, 1993; 2: 98-116.
63. Ueta E, Osaki T, Yoneda K et al. The prevalence of diabetes mellitus in odontogenic infections and oral condidiasis. An analysis of neutrophil suppression. *J Oral Patol Med* 1993: 168-175.

64. Taylor GW. Bidirectional interrelationships between diabetes and periodontal disease: an epidemiological perspective. *Ann Period* 2001; 6: 99-112.
65. Sanz-Sanchez I, Bascones Martinez A.Otras enfermedades periodontales. I:Periodontitis como manifestacion de enfermedades sistematicas. *Av en Periodoncia* 2008; 20 (1): 59-66.
66. Navarro Sanchez AB, Almeida R, Bascones Martinez A. Relacion entre diabetus mellitus y enfermedad periodontal . *Av en Periodoncia* 2002; 14 (1): 9-19.
67. Sanz-Sanchez I, Bascones Martinez A. Diabetus mellitus: Su implication en la patologia oral y periodontal. *Av Odontoestomatol* 2009; 25 (5): 249-263
68. Sanz-Sanchez I, Bascones Martinez A. Diabetus mellitus: Su implication en la patologia oral y periodontal. *Av Odontoestomatol* 2009; 25 (5): 249-263
69. Rodrigo Gomez D. El papel de la genetica en la aparicion y desarrollo de la periodontitis. I: Evidencias cientificans de la asociasion entre periodontitis y genetica. *Av en Periodoncia* 2007;19(2) : 71-81.
70. Riobo Crespo M, Bascones Martinez A. Factores de riesgo de la enfermedad periodontal: factores geneticos. *Av en Periodoncia* 2005; 17 (2): 69-77.
71. Albandar JM. Global risk factors and risk indicators for periodontal disease. Periodontol 2000; 2002; 29: 177-206.
72. Rodrigo Gomez D. El papel de la genetica en la aparicion y desarrollo de la periodontitis. Polimorfismos asociados a la enfermedad periodontal. *Av en Periodoncia* 2008; 20 (2): 121-130.
73. Hassell TM. Genetic influences in caries abd periodontal disease. *Crit Rev Biol Med 1995*; 6: 319- 42.
74. Thomas P. Systemic condicions associated with periodontitis in childhood and adolescence: A review of diagnostic possibilities. *Med Oral Patol Oral Cir Bucal* 2005; 10(2): 142-150.
75. Paters M. The neutrophil disorders. In: Wilson T, Kornman K. The base of periodontology. Medical Pub. Sharov. Sofia 1999. p.. 216-220.
76. Discepoli N, Bascones A. Contraversias etiologicas diagnosticas y terapeuticas de la periodontitis agressiva. *Av en Period* 2008; 20(1):39-40.
77. Rob Bonlter A. A controlled study of relative periodontal attachment loss in people with HIV infection. *J of Period* 2000; 27: 273-6.
78. Glick M. HIV infection . In: Wilson T, Kornman K. The base of periodontology. Medical Pub. Sharov. Sofia 1999. p.. 213-216.

79. Murray PA. Hiv disease as a risk factor for periodontal disease. *Compend Contin Educ Dent* 1994; 15: 1052.
80. Narani N, Epstein JB. Classification of oral lesions in HIV infection. *J of Period* 2001; 28: 137-45.
81. Glick M, Muzyka BC, Salkin LM et al. Necrotizing ulcerative periodontitis. A marker for immune deterioration and a predictor for the diagnosis of AIDS. *J Periodontol* 1994; 65: 393- 397.
82. Smith GLF, Cross DL, Wray D. Comparacion of periodontal disease in HIV seropositive subject and controls. *J of Clin Period* 1995; 22: 558- 68.
83. Robinson PG, Sheiham A, Challacombe SJ et al. The periodontal health of homosexual men with HIV infection. A controlled study. *Oral diseases* 1996; 2: 45- 52.
84. Tezal M, Grossi SG, Ho Aw et al. Alcohol consumption and periodontal disease the NHANES 3. *J Clin Periodontol* 2004; 31: 484.
85. World Health Organization. The World Oral Health Report 2003. http://who/nmh/nmh/orh/03.2.
86. Rose L, Steinberg B. Systemic complication that influence the successful treatment of adult periodontitis. In: Nevis M, Mellonig J. Periodontal therapy. Clinical approaches and evidence of success. Quintessence Publishing Co, Inc. 1998. p.93.
87. Palash T. Adventitious drugs effects. In: Wilson T, Kornman K. The base of periodontology. Medical Pub. Sharov. Sofia 1999. p 219-220.
88. Seymor R. Calcium chanel blockers and gingival overgrowth. *Br Dent J* 1991; 170: 367- 379.
89. Xiao Li, Qingxian L, Xingyu W et al. Nifedipine increase the risk of periodontal disease in subject with Type 2 diabetes mellitus. *J of Period* 2008; 79 (11): 2054-2059.
90. Tsanova S, Tomov G et al. Oral health in patients using drugs. Plovdiv 2011.
91. Moss ME, Beck JD, Kaplan BH et al. Exploratory case- control analysis of psychosocial factors and adult periodontitis. *J Periodontal* 1996; 67: 1060-9.
92. Tabacov N, Grigorov G et al. The prevalence of periodontal diseases among work people in the Combine for non-ferrous metals Plovdiv. *Stomatology* 1992;1:25-28.
93. Rise T. The psychosomatics factors and sress. In: Wilson T, Kornman K. The base of periodontology. Medical Pub. Sharov. Sofia 1999. p 199-200.

94. Barbieri Petrelli G, Mateos Ramirez L. Papel del astres en la etiopatogenia de la enfermedad periodontal. *Av en Period* 2003; 15 (2): 77- 86.
95. Genco RJ, Ho Wa; Grossi SG et al. Relationship of stress distress and inadequate coping behaviors to periodontal disease. *J Periodontol* 1999; 70: 711-23.
96. Deinzer R, Hilpert D, Bach K et al. Effect of academic stress on oral hygiene- a potential link between stress and plaque- associated disease. *J Clin Periodontol* 2001; 28: 459- 64.
97. Rise T. Nutritional deficiencies и metabolic disorders. In: Wilson T, Kornman K. The base of periodontology. Medical Pub. Sharov. Sofia 1999. p 205-208.
98. Nizel A. Role of nutrition in the oral health of the aging patient. *Dent Clin North Am* 1976; 20: 569- 584.
99. Al- Zahrani MS, Bissada NF, Borawskit EA. Obesity and periodontal disease in young, middle-aged and older adults. *J Periodontol* 2003; 74: 610.
100. Saito T, Shimazaki Y, Sakamoto M. Obesity and periodontitis. *N Engl J Med* 1998; 339: 482.
101. Bof de Andiate F. Nutrition and oral health: integral health management for the eldery patient. In: FDI Annual World Dental Congress. 2-5 september 2010. Final Programme: p. 92 - 3 (Abstract Book).
102. Saito T, Koga T et al. Relationship between upper body obesity and periodontitis. J Dent Res 2001; 80: 1631.
103. Wood N, Johnson RB, Streckfus CF. Comparacion of body composition and periodontal disease unit nutritional assessment techniques and NHANES 3. *J Clin Period* 2003; 30: 321.
104. Rose L, Steinberg B. Systemic complication that influence the successful treatment of adult periodontitis. In: Nevis M, Mellonig J. Periodontal therapy. Clinical approaches and evidence of success. Quintessence Publishing Co, Inc. 1998. p.93.
105. Eklund S, Burt B. Risk factors for total tooth loss in US. Longitudinal analysis of national data. *J Pub Heahh Dent* 1994; 54: 5- 14.
106. MacMahon B, Trichopulos D. Epidemiology. Principles and Methods. Little, Brown and Company 1996: p.252.
107. Petersen PE, Ogawa H. Strengthening the prevention of periodontal disease: the WHO approach. J Periodontol 2005; 76:2187-2193.

108. Petersen PE. The Word Oral Health Report 2003:continuous improvement of oral health in 21 century- the approach of the WHO Global Oral Health Programme. Community Dent Oral Epidemiol 2003; 31(1):3-24.
109. Fereira Lopes M, Gusmao E. The impact of chronic periodontitis on quality of life in brazilian subject. *Acta Stomatol Croat* 2009; 43 (2): 89- 98.
110. Caglayan F, Altun O, Miloglu O. Correlation between oral health related quality of life and oral disorders in a turkish patient population. *Med Oral Cir Bucal* 2009; 14 (11): 573- 8.
111. Naito M, Yuasa H, Normura Y. Oral Health status and health related quality of life a systematic review. *J of Oral Science* 2006; 48 (1): 1- 7.
112. Aleksandrova S. Medical ethics. Medical University Pleven Bulgaria 2007.
113. Vodenicharov C, Popova S. Medical ethics. Sofia 2003.
114. Allison PJ, Locker D, Feine GS. Quality of life a dynamic construct. *Social Science and Medicine* 1997; 45:221- 230.
115. Grancharova G, Velcova A et al. Social medicine. Medical University Pleven Bulgaria 2006.
116. Power M. The World Health Organization. Quality of life assessment: development and general psychometric properties. *Social Science and Medicine* 1999; 46 (12): 1569- 89.
117. Allen PF, Mc Millan AS, Walsham D et al. A comparacion of the validity of generic and disease specific measures in the assessment of oral health related quality of life. *Commun Dent Oral Epid* 1999; 27: 344- 352.
118. Broder HL, Slade G, Gaine R et al. Percevied impact of oral health conditions among minority adolescentes. *J Pub Health Dent* 2000; 60: 189- 192.
119. Raphael D, Brown I, Renwick R et al. Quality of life theory and assessment: what are the implications for health promotion. University of Toronto, Centre for Health Promotion., 1994.
120. Inglehart MR, Bagramian RA. Oral health related quality of life. Quintessence Publishing Co, Inc. 2002.
121. Allen PF. Assessment of oral health related quality of life. *Health and quality of life Outcomes* 2003; 1:40.
122. John MT, Micheelis W, Biffar R. Reference values in oral health related quality of life for the abbreviated version of the Oral Health Impact Profile. *Schweiz Monatsschr Zahnmed* 2004; 114 (8): 784- 791.

123. Susan T, Reisine. The social impact of dental disease.Dental Health and Public Policy. *Am J Public Health* 1985; 75: 27- 30.
124. John MT, Koepsell TD, Hujoel P et al. Demographic factors, denture status and oral health related quality of life. *Commun Dent Oral Epidemiol* 2004; 32 (2): 125-132.
125. Raphael D, Brown I, Renwick R. Quality of life theory and assessment:what are the implications for health promotion. Issues in Health promotion series. University of Toronto, Centre for Health Promotion, 1994.
126. Mc Grath C, Bedi R, Gilthorpe MS. Oral health related quality of life: views of the public in the United Kingdom. *Commun Dent Health* 2000; 17: 3-7.
127. Davenport ES, Williams CE et al. Maternal periodontal disease and preterm low birth weight: case- control study. J Dent Res 2002; 81 (5): 313- 8.
128. Karlson E, Lymer U, Hakeberg M. Periodontitis from the patients perspective, a qualitative study. *Int J Dent Higiene* 2009; 7: 23-30.
129. Needleman I, McGrath C, Floyd P. Impact of oral health on the quality of periodontal patients. *J Clin Periodontal* 2004; 31 (6): 457-7.
130. Sam NG, Leung K, Keung W. Oral health related quality of life and periodontal status. *Commun Dent Oral Epidemiology* 2006; 34 (2): 114-122.
131. Drumond Santana T, Costa FO, Zenobio EG. Impact of periodontal disease on quality of life for dentate diabetics. *Cad Saude Pub* 2007; 23(3): 637- 44.
132. Gerritsen A, Finbarr PA, Witter D et al. Tooth loss and Oral health related quality of life: a systematic review and meta-analysis. *Health and Quality of live Outcomes* 2010; 8: 126.
133. Locker D. Disability and disadvantage: The consequences of chronic illness. London Tavistock Publishing 1983.
134. MacEntee MI.The influence of age and gender on oral health and related behavior in an independent eldery population. *Commun Dent Oral Epidemiology* 1993; 21: 234-39.
135. World Health Organization International Statistical Classification of Diseases and Related Problems. Chapter 11 ilnesses of the bucal cavity of the salivary glands and of the maxillary, 10 revision, GenevA WHO; 1992; 524- 37
136. Pearse MA, Thomson WM, Wales AWG. Lifecourse socio- economic mobility and oral health in middle age. *J Dent Res* 2009; 88(10): 938-41.
137. Goldstein R. Chenge your smile. Quintessence Publishing Co, Inc 2009.
138. Ralev R. Frontal aesthetics of the denture. Quintessence BG 1993

139. Georgiev G. Degree of edentulism and removable dental prostheses. Medior Varna Bulgaria 1995.
140. Popov N. Implantology. Publ. Index Sofia Bulgaria 1999.
141. Ritchie CS, Joshipura K, Hung HC. Nutrition as a mediator in the relation between oral and systematic disease: associations between specific measures of adult ooral health and nutrition outcomes. *Crit Rev Oral Biol Med* 2002; 13: 291.
142. Millwood J, Heath MR. Food choice by older people.The use of semi-structured interviews with open and closed questions. *Geradontology* 2000; 17: 25- 32.
143. Buirt BA. Epidemiology of dental diseases in the elderly. *Clin Geriat Med* 1992; 8: 447- 59.
144. Locker D: Social and psychological consequences of oral disorders. *In: Turning strategy into action (Edited by: Kay EJ)*. Manchester: Eden Bianchipress 1995.
145. Fitzpatrick R, Fletcher A, Gore D,et al : Quality of life measures in health care. I: Application and issues in assessment. *BMJ* 1992 , 305:1074-1077.
146. Slade G, Spencer A: Development and evaluation of the Oral Health Impact Profile. *Community Dent Health* 1994, 11:3-11.
147. Scaret E, Astrom A.: Oral health related quality of life . http://egohid.eu/Documents/OralHealth-relatedQualityofLife.pdf.
148. Allen P, McMillan A, Locker D: An assessment of the responsiveness of the Oral Health Impact Profile in a clinical trial. *Comm Dent Oral Epidemiol* 2001 , 29:175-182.
149. Bowling A: Measuring disease. *A review of disease specific quality of life measurement scales* Buckingham: Open University Press 1995.
150. Cohen L, Jago J: Toward formulation of socio-dental indicators. *International Journal of Health Services* 1976, 6:681-698.
151. Reisine S: Dental disease and work loss. *J Dent Res* 1984, 63:1158-1161.
152. Reisine S: Dental health and public policy: The social impact of dental disease. *Am J Public Health* 1985 , 74:27-30.
153. Bergner M, Bobbit B, Carter W, et al: The Sickness Impact Profile: Development and final revision of a health status measure. *Medical Care* 1981, 19: 787-805.
154. Nikias M: Oral disease and the quality of life. *Am J Public Health* 1985, 75:11-12

155. Locker D: Measuring oral health: A conceptual framework. *Community Dental Health* 1988, 5:3-18.
156. Atchison K, Dolan T: Development of the Geriatric Oral Health Assessment Index. *J Dent Educ* 1990, 54:680-687.
157. Locker D, Miller Y: Evaluation of subjective oral health status indicators. *J Public Health Dent* 1994, 54:167-176.
158. Wolinsky F, Wolinsky S. Background attitudinal and behavioral patterns of individuals occupying eight discrete health states. *Sociol Health Illness* 1981; 3:31-48.
159. Cushing A, Sheiham A, Maizels J. Developing socio-dental indicators. The social impact of dental disease. *Community Dental Health* 1986; 3:3-17.
160. Elinson J. In: Socio-medical health indicators. Elinson J. and Siegmann A, Eds. Farringdale: Baywood Pub Inc. 1979:3-7.
161. Heydecke G, Locker D et al. Oral and general health related quality of life with conventional and implant dentures. Commun Dentistry and Oral Epidemiology 2003; 31: 161-8.
162. Davenport ES, Williams CE et al. Maternal periodontal disease and preterm low birth weight: case- control study. J Dent Res 2002; 81 (5): 313- 8.
163. Locker D: Issues in measuring change in self-perceived oral health status. *Comm Dent Oral Epidemiol* 1998, 26:41-47.
164. Loureiro A, Costa F et al. The impact of periodontal disease on the quality of life of individuas with Down syndrome. Oral Health 2007; 12: 1.
165. Bobetsis YA, Barros SP, Offenbacher S. Exploring the relationship between periodontal disease and pregnancy complications. *J Am Dent Assoc* 2006; 2 (137): 75- 135.
166. Wandera M.; Astrom A; Engebretsen I. Peridontal status; tooth loss and self-reported periodontal problems effects on oral impacts on daily performances; OIDS in pregnant women in Uganda. *Health and quality of life outcomes* 2009; 7:89
167. Astrom A, Okullo I. Validity and realibity of the OIDP frequency scale: a cross-sectional study of adolescencets in Uganda. BMC Oral Health 2003; 3:5.
168. Meas F, Wright P. Oral Health Impact on Daily Performance in Patients with implant stabilized overdenturesand patients with conventional complete dentures. QUIntessence J Oral Maxillofac Implants 2001; 16: 700- 712.
169. Leao A, Sheiham A: The development of a socio-dental measure of Dental Impacts on Daily Living *Community Dental Health* 1996, 13:22-26

170. Stoykova M. Cancer of oral cavity and jowl- epidemiology, quality of life and social rehabilitation. Medical University Plovdiv Bulgaria 2006 (Disertation)
171. Locker D, Slade G: Oral health and quality of life among older adults: the Oral Health Impact Profile. *J Can Dent Ass* 1993; 59:830-844.
172. Slade G, Spencer A, Locker D, et al: Variations in the social impact of oral conditions among older adults in South Australia, Ontario, and North Carolina. *J Dent Res* 1996, 75:1439-1450.
173. Leao A, Sheiham A: Relation between clinical dental status and subjective impacts on daily living. *J Dent Res* 1995, 74:1408-1413.
174. Kressin N: Associations among different assessments of oral healthoutcomes. *J Dent Educ* 1996, 60:501-507.
175. Sheiham A, Steele J, Marcenes W, et al: Prevalence of impacts of dental and oral disorders and their effects on eating among older people; a national survey in Great Britain. *Comm Dent Oral Epidemiol* 2001 28:195-203
176. Allison P, Locker D, Jokovic A, et al: A Cross-cultural Study of Oral Health Values. *J Dent Res* 1999, 78:643-649
177. Araujo AC, Gusmao ES, Batista JE. Impact of periodontal disease on quality of life. Quintessence Int. 2010; 41 (6): 111-8
178. Shanbhag S, Dahiya M, Croucher R. The impact of periodontal therapy on oral health-related quality of life in adults. J Clin Periodontol 2012; 39(8):725-35.
179. Ritchie CS, Joshipura K, Hung HC. Nutrition as a mediator in the relation between oral and systematic disease: associations between specific measures of adult ooral health and nutrition outcomes. Crit Rev Oral Biol Med 2002; 13: 291.
180. Millwood J, Heath MR. Food choice by older people.The use of semi-structured interviews with open and closed questions. Geradontology 2000; 17: 25- 32.
181. Sheiham A, Steele J, Marcenes W, et al: Prevalence of impacts of dental and oral disorders and their effects on eating among older people; a national survey in Great Britain. Comm Dent Oral Epidemiol 2001 28:195-203
182. Chambrone LA, Chambrone L. Tooth loss in well-maintained patients with chronic periodontit during long-term supportive therapy in Brazil. J Clin Period 2006; 33(10):759-764.

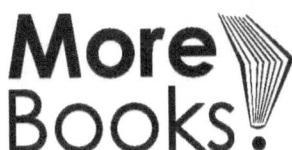
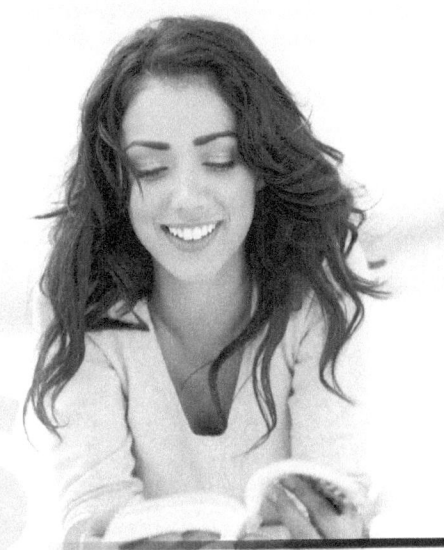

I want morebooks!

Buy your books fast and straightforward online - at one of the world's fastest growing online book stores! Environmentally sound due to Print-on-Demand technologies.

Buy your books online at
www.get-morebooks.com

Kaufen Sie Ihre Bücher schnell und unkompliziert online – auf einer der am schnellsten wachsenden Buchhandelsplattformen weltweit!
Dank Print-On-Demand umwelt- und ressourcenschonend produziert.

Bücher schneller online kaufen
www.morebooks.de

OmniScriptum Marketing DEU GmbH
Heinrich-Böcking-Str. 6-8
D - 66121 Saarbrücken
Telefax: +49 681 93 81 567-9

info@omniscriptum.com
www.omniscriptum.com

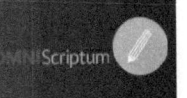

www.ingramcontent.com/pod-product-compliance
Lightning Source LLC
Chambersburg PA
CBHW031547210526
45464CB00003B/1183